Your No-Nonsense Guide to

Eating Well

By Maeve Hanan
Registered Dietitian

First published in June 2020

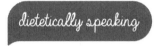

Copyright © 2020 Dietetically Speaking
(Maeve Hanan, Registered Dietitian)

ISBN: 979-8-6468-9128-1

The information included in this book is not intended to replace
individualised advice you have received from your GP or another
healthcare professional. If in doubt, always seek support from a
medical professional in relation to your health. The author and
contributors disclaim any liability, directly or indirectly, from the use
of the material in this book by any individual. The content of this
book is targeted at healthy adults, rather than those who have
additional nutritional needs — such as athletes or those with medical
conditions. This book is not intended to be used by those under the
age of 18. Most of the guidelines referenced in this book are from
Ireland and the UK.

A massive thank you to Anthony O'Neill, Zachary Wenger, Alex Larkin, Alison Thompson, Robin Hanan and Kathleen Connolly for their help with this book.

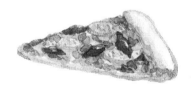

3

About Dietetically Speaking

My name is Maeve Hanan and I am a Registered Dietitian from Ireland. I have a background in clinical nutrition, having worked in the National Health Service in the UK as a General Dietitian (working in the hospital and in out-patient clinics), a Stroke Specialist Dietitian and a Paediatric Specialist Dietitian. I also have a variety of experience in nutrition consultancy and nutrition communication — including health writing, working with the media and creating content for social media. I currently work as a Consultant Dietitian, providing nutrition consultancy services and seeing clients in private practice.

I created Dietetically Speaking in September 2015 because I was feeling extremely frustrated about the abundance of nutritional nonsense I was seeing in the news and on social media. My aim has always been to spread evidence-based nutrition messages, debunk nutritional nonsense and to promote a way of eating that is healthy, enjoyable and realistic.

Over the years I have worked with many people who feel that eating well is a daunting, tedious, confusing or time-consuming task. So I am very passionate about demystifying eating well, and demonstrating how achievable this can be.

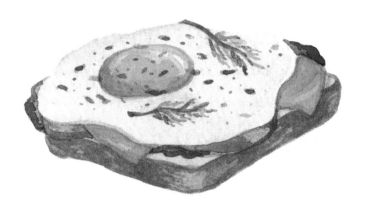

Introduction

This book draws on my experience of working with countless clients who feel motivated to eat well, but at the same time find this to be a daunting task. This is understandable considering how much confusion surrounds nutritional advice, how busy our lives have become and how common it is to fall into the 'food perfectionist' trap. I was also inspired to write this book by my own journey with food, as I want to help others to find a way of eating that is balanced, satisfying and realistic.

Before we delve into my tips and meal ideas, it is important to explain what 'eating well' means. I define eating well as enjoying a variety of foods in sufficient quantities to support good health and happiness. Eating well is not just about the food itself; it includes our enjoyment of food and developing a healthy relationship with food. I prefer this term to 'healthy eating' as it allows more flexibility, and flexibility is a key aspect of a balanced approach to eating. Eating well is often associated with trying to lose weight. Although weight loss can occur as a side effect of eating well in some cases, losing weight is not the focus of this book. My approach to eating well focuses on the bigger picture of overall health, rather than the pursuit of weight loss.

This book is for everyone who feels overwhelmed by trying to eat well. My aim is to demystify and simplify this process, because eating well should not become a source of unnecessary stress and unhappiness.

This book begins by outlining my top ten nutrition tips and then takes you step by step through advice for food shopping, meal preparation and creating balanced meals and snacks. Chapter 6 explains the importance of adopting the mindset of a 'food realist' rather than a 'food perfectionist'. The second half of the book contains 50 quick and balanced meal ideas, so that you can take the advice from this book and translate it into nutritious meals on your plate.

As you will learn throughout this book, my philosophy is that food should compliment your life, not dominate it. I strongly believe in this message because food can add so much enjoyment to our lives, as well as fuelling our body so that we can do the activities that we love. Eating well should be a form of self-care, so this should not become stressful, obsessive or restrictive.

I hope you enjoy this book and that it provides you with the tools to eat well for long-term health and wellbeing.

If you enjoy this book or if you have any feedback, please let me know:

Instagram:	@dieteticallyspeaking
Twitter:	@DieteticSpeak
Email:	maeve@dieteticallyspeaking.com

CONTENTS

Breakfast Options

Lunch Options

Dinner Options

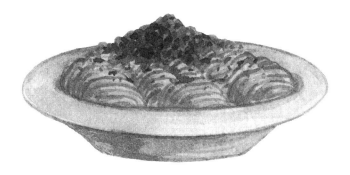

Chapter 1

Ten No-Nonsense Nutrition Tips

Understanding the main principles of eating well is extremely useful and empowering. This helps you to simplify nutritional advice, and to filter out the nutritional nonsense you will inevitably encounter. To guide you through these principles, I have divided this chapter into ten evidence-based nutrition tips.

1. Consume plenty of high-fibre, plant-based foods

Examples: Fruit, vegetables, beans, chickpeas, lentils, peas, nuts, seeds, oats, quinoa, wholegrain couscous, bulgur wheat, freekeh, pearl barley, wholegrain bread and wholegrain pasta.

Health benefits: Consuming about 30g of fibre per day from a variety of plant-based sources is extremely important for our gut health.[1-3] This has been found to normalise bowel movements, reduce the risk of constipation, feed beneficial gut bacteria and increase the production of short-chain fatty acids (SCFAs).[1-2] SCFAs provide energy for the cells in our colon and are thought to have a number of health benefits, such as reducing inflammation.[2] Consuming enough fibre is also filling and is associated with a lower risk of bowel cancer, heart disease and type 2 diabetes.[2] These plant-based foods also provide a number of other essential nutrients. For example, many fruit and vegetables contain vitamin C, folate, beta-carotene (a form of vitamin A) and vitamin K. Similarly, wholegrains, nuts and seeds are good sources of B vitamins, vitamin E, iron and zinc.

Additional tips: We are advised to eat a few portions of wholegrains and at least five portions of fruit and vegetables every day. So aim to include these high-fibre foods at most of your meals and snacks. Chapter 4 contains advice on portion sizes, and I have included plenty of high-fibre recipes in the second half of this book. Where possible, try to wash fruit and vegetables rather than peeling them in order to maintain their fibre content. When increasing your intake of fibre, it is important to stay well hydrated and to add in high-fibre foods gradually so that your gut has time to adjust.

2. Include a high-protein food with every meal

Examples: Meat, poultry, fish, shellfish, eggs, dairy, beans, lentils, chickpeas, mycoprotein (such as Quorn[TM]), seitan, tofu, tempeh and other soya-based foods such as soya milk, soya yogurt, soya-based mince or vegetarian sausages.

Health benefits: Protein is essential for skin health and wound healing, as well as maintaining healthy bone and muscle mass.[4] It is also a very filling nutrient and a building block for important hormones and enzymes.[4] These high-protein foods also provide a number of other vital nutrients. For example, many of the foods listed above are high in iron. Meat, fish, eggs and dairy are also great sources of vitamin B12 which is needed by our nervous system and for red blood cell formation, DNA creation and releasing energy from food. Milk and yogurt are also excellent sources of iodine, which is essential for healthy thyroid function.

Additional tips: Adding a high-protein food to a snack can make this more filling and satisfying. Chapter 5 provides examples of snack combinations, and Chapter 4 outlines suggested portion sizes of high-protein foods.

3. Consume mainly unsaturated fats

Examples: Olive oil, rapeseed oil, sunflower oil, nuts, seeds, avocado, hummus and pesto (made with olive oil).

Health benefits: Replacing foods that are high in saturated and trans fat (such as fried foods, butter, pastries, etc.), with foods high in unsaturated fat helps to keep our cholesterol at a healthy level.[5] Dietary fats also provide energy, play a role in hormone production and help us to absorb vitamin A, D, E and K from our food.

Additional tips: Although fats play an important role in our diet, we generally need smaller quantities of high-fat foods as compared to other food groups — as outlined in Chapter 4.

4. Eat at least three portions of high-calcium foods per day

Examples: Milk, yogurt, cheese, calcium-fortified plant-based milk or yogurt, sardines (with bones), tofu, tahini, kale, bok choy and chickpeas.

<u>Health benefits</u>: Calcium is an essential building block of our bones and teeth. This mineral also plays an important role in blood clotting, muscle contraction and nerve transmission.[6]

<u>Additional tips</u>: Children and teenagers aged 9-18, along with pregnant, breastfeeding and post-menopausal women are advised to consume five portions of high-calcium foods per day (whereas most adults require three portions per day).[3] You can find advice on portion sizes for high-calcium foods in Chapter 4 — for example, a 200ml glass of milk, a 125g pot of yogurt or two thumbs of cheese (roughly 25g) each count as one portion of calcium. Please note: a cup of chickpeas, a tablespoon of tahini or a cup of steamed bok choy only count as half a portion of calcium.

5. Regularly consume iron-rich foods

<u>Examples</u>: Red meat, liver, egg yolks, poultry, seafood, beans, nuts, seeds, iron-fortified cereals, dried apricots, spirulina and green leafy vegetables such as spinach and swiss chard.

<u>Health benefits</u>: Iron is needed by the body to form haemoglobin in red blood cells, which transports oxygen around the body.[7] Therefore, a lack of this vital mineral can lead to iron deficiency anaemia and symptoms such as tiredness and shortness of breath. Iron is also important for a healthy immune system.[7]

<u>Additional tips</u>: One to three portions of red meat per week can be included in a healthy diet. Processed red meat like sausages, ham, bacon and salami should only be consumed occasionally. Pregnant women should avoid liver and pâté as

these foods are very high in vitamin A, which can be harmful to an unborn baby. The type of iron found in plant-based foods like green leafy vegetables (non-haem iron) is not absorbed as well as iron from animal-based foods like red meat (haem iron). However, you can increase non-haem iron absorption by consuming vitamin C along with this, such as a small glass of orange juice or a handful of strawberries, chopped red pepper or broccoli. Whereas, drinking tea or coffee within an hour of eating an iron-rich food has been found to reduce iron absorption.

6. Eat at least one portion of oily fish and one portion of white fish every week

Examples of oily fish: Salmon, mackerel, trout, herring, sardines and kippers.

Examples of white fish: Cod, sea bass, sea bream, haddock, plaice, pollock, coley, halibut and red mullet.

Health benefits: Fish is a nutritious food as it contains protein and a number of important vitamins and minerals. For example, cod and haddock are great sources of iodine. Oily fish is an excellent source of omega-3 fatty acids — which play a vital role in our heart, brain and eye health.[8] Studies have found that consuming oily fish at least once per week is associated with a lower risk of heart disease.[9] Taking an omega-3 supplement can be useful in some cases, but this is generally not as good for our health as compared to eating oily fish.[9-10]

Additional tips: Those who don't eat oily fish should consume plant-based sources of omega-3 every day. Examples include: rapeseed oil, flaxseed oil, walnuts, flaxseeds or chia seeds. This group may also benefit from taking an omega-3 supplement which is made from algae. However, the jury is still out on how effective these supplements are in the long term.[11] If in doubt, please seek individual advice from a Dietitian — this is especially important for high-risk groups like pregnant women, breastfeeding women, infants and children. To limit exposure to pollutants which can be found in fish, women who are pregnant, breastfeeding or trying for a baby are advised to avoid shark, swordfish and marlin. They are also advised to limit their intake of oily fish to two 140g portions per week and to consume no more than four tins of tuna (140g when drained) or two tuna steaks per week. Pregnant women also need to avoid fish liver oil supplements, as these can contain dangerously high levels of vitamin A for a developing baby.

7. Consume smaller amounts of foods that are high in saturated fat, salt and sugar

Examples: Biscuits, chocolate, cake, crisps, pastries, pies, chips, fried food, butter, coconut oil, salted crackers and salted nuts.

Health benefits: Although there is no need to avoid these 'sometimes foods' completely, it is best to eat them in smaller amounts in order to optimise our health. For example, a high intake of saturated fat and salt is bad for our heart, and regularly consuming sugary foods and drinks is bad for our teeth.[2]

8. Consider taking a vitamin D supplement during winter if you don't live close to the equator

Examples: Vitamin D spray, tablets or capsules.

Rationale: Studies have found that our skin cannot produce vitamin D during the winter months in countries which are situated 37 degrees or more above or below the equator — as highlighted on the image below.[12-13] For this reason, we are advised to consider taking a 10 microgram vitamin D supplement from October to March.[13] In addition, people who have limited sun exposure in the summer months may benefit from taking this supplement all year round. For example, being housebound, or regularly wearing sunscreen reduces exposure to the type of UV rays which lead to vitamin D production in the skin. It is generally difficult to get enough vitamin D from our diet, unless you consume a lot of products which are fortified with vitamin D.

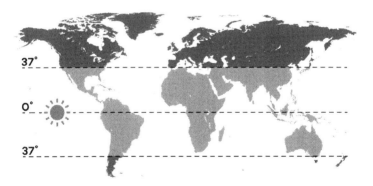

Health benefits: Vitamin D is needed for the absorption of calcium and phosphorus, so it plays an essential role in maintaining healthy bones and teeth.[13] Vitamin D is also important for promoting muscle strength, immune function and balancing inflammation levels.[13-14]

9. Healthy hydration

Examples: Water, milk, fortified plant-based milk, tea, coffee, 150ml of fruit juice or shop-bought smoothie once per day.

Rationale: Water is usually the best drink to consume. Milk or fortified plant-based milks are also good choices to include a few times per day. Out of the various plant-based milks on offer, soya is generally the most nutritious option as it has the highest protein content. 150ml of fruit juice or shop-bought smoothie can count as one portion of fruit once per day, however, anything above this counts towards our daily sugar intake. Homemade smoothies can count as more than one portion of fruit or vegetables as they contain more fibre than most shop-bought versions. Tea and coffee count towards your daily fluid intake, but it is advised to limit our caffeine intake to three to four average cups of tea or coffee per day.[15] Drinking too much alcohol is dehydrating and is associated with a higher risk of numerous diseases, including liver disease, heart disease and certain types of cancer.[16] Therefore, we are advised to limit our alcohol intake to 14 units per week and to have at least two alcohol-free days per week.[16] One unit of alcohol is approximately half a pint of 4% beer, half a medium glass of 13% wine or 25ml of spirits.[16] Similarly, if sugary drinks are consumed, this should only be occasional. Pregnant women are advised to avoid alcohol and to consume no more than 200mg of caffeine per day (which is about two cups of instant coffee or three cups of tea).

Health benefits: Fluid makes up about 50-60% of the human body.[17] This has a number of important functions such as removing waste, temperature regulation, joint lubrication, transporting nutrients and maintaining kidney health.[18] Dehydration can lead to fatigue, trouble concentrating, constipation and headaches. Adults need at least eight glasses or cups (1600ml) of fluid per day, but this depends on body size, physical activity level and how hot the environment is.[18] A great way to check your hydration level is to look at the colour of your urine — if this is a pale yellow colour it means that you are well hydrated, darker urine indicates that you need to drink more fluid.

10. Embrace variety and flexibility

Examples: Mix it up by eating different types of fruit, vegetables, pulses, grains, nuts, seeds, and sources of protein. Make sure that you 'eat the rainbow' by consuming lots of different coloured fruit and vegetables. Also, allow yourself to enjoy 'sometimes foods' in moderation (like chocolate, biscuits, crisps, chips, etc.).

Health benefits: Consuming a varied diet provides a wide range of nutrients and is usually a satisfying and enjoyable way of eating. As well as this, evidence is emerging about the benefits of a varied diet in terms of optimising our gut health, particularly when consuming a variety of plant-based foods.[1] Flexibility is a key part of a varied and balanced diet, so no food needs to be completely off-limits — unless you are allergic to it of course. Eating is also an important part of many social occasions, and socialising is linked with numerous health benefits, such as improvements in mental health, brain function and immunity.[19-21] So being too rigid with dietary choices can get in the way of enjoying food with loved ones or at times of celebration. Chapter 6 contains more information about adopting a flexible and healthy mindset in terms of food choice.

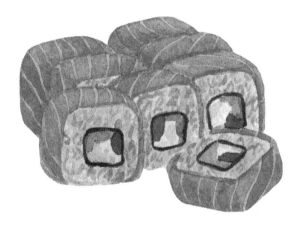

Chapter 2

Food Shopping

Food shopping is a dreaded task for many people, but having the right food available at home is a key step in the process of eating well.

Here are my top three tips for hassle-free food shopping:

1. Be prepared and make a list before you go — this can be a paper list, a note on your phone or you can try using a checklist app.
2. If you are regularly short on time, you can try booking supermarket deliveries online. Once you do one online shop most supermarkets save your list so it's really quick to make a few changes the next time you make an order.
3. Stock up on staple foods (as listed below) so that you can easily throw together quick and balanced meals.

Shopping List Staples:

You can use the following lists as a guide for creating a balanced shopping list. You don't need to include everything listed below on your shopping list, and of course you can add in other foods which you enjoy, but you should include some foods from each of the food groups.

Fruit and vegetables:
- Frozen fruit, e.g. berries or tropical mixed fruit
- Tinned fruit, e.g. peaches or pineapple (in juice or water rather than syrup, drain the juice or water before eating)
- Frozen vegetables, e.g. spinach, mushrooms, chopped onion, butternut squash, peas or stir-fry vegetable mixes
- Tinned vegetables, e.g. sweetcorn or tomatoes
- Fresh fruit, vegetables and salad options
- Dried fruit, e.g. raisins, sultanas, dates, dried apricots or dried figs
- Tomato or garlic purée (or fresh tomato and garlic)

High-protein foods:
- Fresh or frozen meat, fish, shellfish, chicken or turkey
- Frozen bean burgers or mycoprotein (e.g. Quorn™)
- Tinned fish, e.g. tuna, mackerel or salmon
- Pre-cooked fillets of salmon, mackerel or chicken
- Smoked salmon or mackerel
- Tinned or dried pulses, e.g. beans, chickpeas or lentils
- Tofu or tempeh
- Dairy or soya-based dairy alternatives, e.g. milk and yogurt

Carbohydrates:
- Oats
- Wholegrain breakfast cereals, e.g. wheat biscuit cereal or low-sugar muesli
- Oatcakes or rye crispbreads
- Wholegrain bread, pitta or wraps

- Wholegrain pasta or noodles
- Dried rice, quinoa, couscous or bulgur wheat
- Microwave bags of rice or mixed grains (quinoa, bulgur wheat, etc.)
- Potatoes or sweet potatoes

Fats:
- Hummus
- Avocado or guacamole
- Pesto (made with olive oil)
- Cheese
- Mixed nuts
- Mixed seeds
- Nut butter, e.g. peanut, almond or cashew butter
- Tahini
- Vegetable oil, e.g. olive, rapeseed, sunflower or avocado oil
- Olive-based spread or butter

Other:
- Dried or fresh herbs and spices.
- Ready meals can be useful for when you are short on time or energy, e.g. vegetable lasagne, bean soup, cottage pie or fish pie. Try to mainly choose products that contain less salt, saturated fat and sugar. You can also boost the nutritional content of the meal by adding extra vegetables or a side salad.
- Smaller amounts of 'sometimes food or drinks' for enjoyment, e.g. chocolate, biscuits, crisps or alcohol.

Reading Food Labels

It can be confusing to know which products to buy, as there are so many different brands and food products available.

Tips for reading food labels (based on current EU food label law):[22]

1. Terms like 'natural', 'organic', or 'diet' don't necessarily mean that a product is the healthiest option; it is better to look at the ingredients list and nutritional content.

2. Ingredients are listed in order from high to low e.g. if sugar is the first ingredient on the list, then sugar is the main ingredient.

3. On the back of the packet, the nutritional content is usually listed per 100g and per suggested serving size. However, some labels will only list the 'per 100g' nutrition information.

4. If a product has a traffic light label on the front, this gives a quick snapshot of calorie content per serving, as well as the fat, saturated fat, sugar and salt content (see image below):
    • Green means low, i.e. a healthier choice
    • Amber means medium, i.e. fine to consume most of the time
    • Red means high, i.e. it should be eaten less often

6. When interpreting the per 100g nutritional values on the back of the label (see image below):
   - Sugar: 5g or less is low, more than 22.5g is high
   - Salt: 0.3g or less is low, more than 1.5g is high
   - Saturated fat: 1.5g or less is low, more than 5g is high
   - Fibre: 6g or higher means high in fibre

	Fat	Saturated Fat	Sugars	Salt
High per 100g	Over 17.5g	Over 5g	Over 22.5g	Over 1.5g
Medium per 100g	Between 3.1g and 17.5g	Between 1.6g and 5g	Between 5.1g and 22.5g	Between 0.4g and 1.5g
Low per 100g	3g and below	1.5g and below	5g and below	0.3g and below

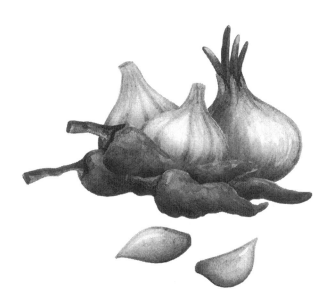

Chapter 3

Meal Preparation

Lacking the time, energy or motivation to prepare a meal are common barriers to eating well. So this chapter outlines time-saving tips for meal preparation.

1. Stock up on nutritious convenience food

Having ingredients to hand which can be quickly transformed into a balanced meal or snack is half the battle.

Some of my favourite nutritious convenience foods include:
- Frozen fruit and vegetables
- Tinned beans, lentils, chickpeas and tomatoes
- Tomato and garlic purée
- Dried herbs and spices
- Milk and yogurt
- Sliced or grated cheese
- Eggs
- Couscous
- Tinned fish
- Pre-cooked fish and chicken
- Pre-pressed tofu
- Wholegrain bread, pitta, wraps and crackers
- Pouches of pre-cooked grains (such as rice, couscous, quinoa, bulgur wheat, etc.)
- Wholegrain pasta and noodles
- Oats

- Nuts, seeds and nut butter
- Hummus
- Olive oil

Take a look at the shopping list suggestions in Chapter 2 for more ideas.

2. Make use of your microwave

It is a myth that it is unhealthy or unsafe to prepare food in the microwave. In fact, microwaving vegetables can often preserve more nutrients when compared with other cooking methods, such as boiling.[23] Microwaving is also an extremely convenient way of reheating leftovers and preparing meals in minutes, such as: porridge, scrambled eggs and beans.

Tips for microwaving:
- It is important to use microwave-safe containers.
- Make sure your microwave is functioning properly and that the seal around the door is not damaged.
- Try using a microwave steamer to steam fish, vegetables and potatoes.
- When reheating leftovers, make sure that the food is piping hot in the middle before eating.
- To make sure food is evenly heated: microwave the food for a few minutes, take it out and stir it, then microwave for another few minutes — this is particularly important when reheating rice.[24]
- To stop leftovers from drying out while microwaving, you can place a small glass of water (in a microwave-safe glass) in the centre of the dish.

3. Time-saving kitchen hacks

- Make use of your kitchen scissors: This is one of my favourite time-saving cooking hacks. I use kitchen scissors to chop spring onion, broccoli heads, fresh herbs, fresh mozzarella and smoked salmon.
- Try an egg slicer: This can be used to quickly chop soft fruit and vegetables such as strawberries, peeled kiwi, mushroom, avocado, courgette and cooked potato.
- 'One-pot' meals: This is a great way of saving on the washing up! Examples of one-pot meals include risottos, stews and curries. The following recipes which are included at the end of this book can be made in one pot: chilli beef hash, chicken and chickpea curry, lentil and butterbean stew, lentil and vegetable soup, tofu and sweet potato satay, bean chilli and lentil bolognese.
- Slow-cooked meals: If you have a slow cooker, this can also be a handy way of preparing meals like stews and casseroles. Although you do need to plan and prepare the food in advance if you are using a slow cooker.
- Make frozen flavour cubes: These can be prepared in advance to save time at a later date. Chop and sauté onion and garlic in olive oil, then freeze this cooked mixture (encased in olive oil) in an ice cube tray. You can then pop it straight from the freezer into the pan when you need it. Another option is to add fresh herbs and olive oil straight into an ice cube tray and freeze.

4. Cook in bulk

This is one of the best things you can do for saving time, effort and money when it comes to cooking. So get in the habit of cooking extras as often as you can by doubling or tripling recipes. Then you can either freeze the leftovers or keep them in the fridge for lunch or dinner the next day.

Make sure to follow food safety advice when freezing and reheating food:[24]

- Check the star rating on your freezer to see how long you can safely freeze food for, this usually ranges from one week to six months.
- Frozen food can be covered and defrosted in the fridge overnight. It is best to place this on the bottom shelf of the fridge to avoid contaminating other food (otherwise juices from defrosting meat, chicken or fish can drip onto other foods).
- If you are defrosting food using the microwave you should cook the food immediately afterwards — check your microwave's handbook for specific guidelines.
- Don't refreeze defrosted food unless it has first been cooked to over 70°C for at least two minutes (in this case it should only be refrozen once).

You can find updated information about safely storing, cooking and reheating food on the Food Safety Authority website.

At the end of this book, I have included lots of recipes for meals which are suitable for bulk cooking and freezing. For example, my chicken and chickpea curry, butterbean stew, bean chilli, lentil and vegetable soup, Mexican bean soup and lentil bolognese.

5. Make adaptable dishes

This handy approach means that you can enjoy a variety of meals, with much less effort involved compared with cooking entirely separate dishes. This is particularly good for people who get tired of eating the same meal for a few days in a row when you have prepared a batch of meals. This involves making a big batch of one dish and then making slight adaptations so that this can be incorporated into different dishes.

For example, a batch of chilli can be:
- Served with rice
- Used as a burrito filling
- Made into a quesadilla
- Served on a baked potato
- Made into Mexican bean soup (you can find this recipe in the meal ideas section of this book)

Similarly, a batch of lentil and vegetable soup can be:
- Blended and used as a pasta sauce
- Made into a curry by adding some curry powder and serving with rice
- Made into a lentil bake (you can find this recipe in the meal ideas section at the end of this book)

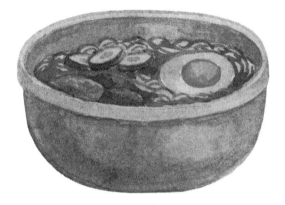

Chapter 4

Creating Meals

Consuming balanced meals most of the time is important for our health. This chapter shows you how to create nutritious and satisfying meals which provide lasting energy. This is a general guideline, so if you have any additional nutritional needs please seek support from a Registered Dietitian.

It is also important to allow yourself to have some flexibility with this. For example, some people like to follow the '80:20 approach' by aiming to balance their meals in this way roughly 80% of the time and enjoying 'sometimes foods' (like chocolate, takeaways, etc.) roughly 20% of the time.

Balancing Your Plate

As outlined in the image below, a balanced meal can be created by combining:

- Plenty of fruit and vegetables — to fill roughly half of your plate. Aim to 'eat the rainbow' by eating lots of different types of fruit and vegetables, in a variety of colours.
- High-protein food — to fill roughly a quarter of your plate. Examples include meat, poultry, fish, eggs, dairy, beans, pulses, tofu or other soya-based foods such as tempeh, soya mince, soya milk or soya yogurt.

- Starchy carbohydrates — to fill roughly a quarter of your plate. Such as potato, cereals, pasta, rice, oats, couscous, quinoa, bulgur wheat or bread (ideally wholegrain versions).
- Smaller amounts of healthy fats — such as nuts, seeds, avocado, hummus, olive oil, sunflower oil or rapeseed oil.

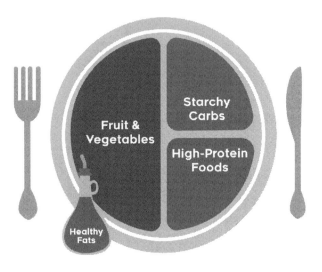

You can find 50 examples of balanced meal ideas at the end of this book.

Although this is a general guide for creating a balanced meal, remember that it is fine to add some extras for taste and enjoyment. For example, you may enjoy having a dessert a few times per week, or adding some honey or chocolate to a bowl of porridge. Chapter 6 contains more information about this.

Portion Sizes

Average nutritional requirements used as daily 'reference intakes' on food labels are usually based on the needs of a 60kg woman, these are:[25]

- Energy: 2,000 kcal
- Total fat: less than 70g
- Saturated fat: less than 20g
- Carbohydrate: at least 260g
- Total sugars: 90g (including 30g of free sugars per day i.e. honey, syrups and sugar which is added to food and drink)
- Protein: 50g
- Salt: less than 6g

However, nutritional requirements and the portion sizes needed to achieve these are very individual and can vary a lot between people, depending on factors like body size, activity levels and sex.

The balanced meal plate image on the previous page and the 'handy portion sizes' image on the next page can be used as a rough guide for estimating your portion sizes.

Handy Portion Sizes

Starchy Carbohydrates:
Fist-sized Portion

Fruit & Vegetables:
Two Handfuls

Cheese, Oil & Nut Butter:
Two Thumbs

Red Meat, Tofu, Nuts & Seeds:
Palm-sized Portion

Chicken & Fish:
Hand-sized Portion

Butter & Sugar:
Tip of the Thumb

Other examples of standard portion sizes include:

- A 200ml glass of milk (or calcium-fortified plant-based milk)
- A 125mg pot or 3 tablespoons of yogurt (or calcium-fortified plant-based yogurt)
- Two eggs
- Half of a 400g tin of beans
- Two slices of bread
- One large pitta or wrap
- Two medium potatoes
- One nest of noodles

Rather than focusing on specific portion sizes, some people prefer to be guided by their feelings of hunger and fullness, as per the Intuitive Eating approach.[26] Different approaches suit different people, so see what works best for you or speak to a registered nutrition professional for individual advice.

Chapter 5

Choosing Snacks

Although snacking too frequently throughout the day can put us off our meals, snacks can absolutely be included in a healthy diet. Some people don't feel the need for any snacks, whereas others find that having two or three snacks per day works well for them — as outlined in the sample meal pattern below. The urge to snack can also vary day to day, depending on what you have eaten recently, how well you have slept, how active you have been, your mood and changes in your hormone levels etc.

Sample daily meal pattern:

Breakfast
Optional snack
Lunch
Optional snack
Dinner
Optional snack

A good rule of thumb for creating a nutritious and satisfying snack is to combine a plant-based food with a portion of high-protein food. For example, combining a portion of fruit, vegetables or a wholegrain food with nuts, seeds, cheese, milk or yogurt (or soya-based milk or yogurt). Take a look at the following snack ideas for more examples of snack combinations.

As discussed in Chapter 4 and Chapter 6, it is healthy to approach these guidelines in a flexible way. So don't feel guilty for having 'sometimes foods' as an occasional snack, such as biscuits, chocolate or crisps.

Snack ideas:

- A piece of fruit and a handful of nuts
- A small pot of natural or greek yogurt and a handful of berries
- A handful of mixed nuts and dried fruit
- A piece of fruit and a tablespoon of nut butter
- A handful of roasted chickpeas or edamame beans with paprika and a handful of dried fruit
- A handful of cherry tomatoes and a falafel
- Sliced carrots, peppers, cucumber or sugar snap peas and a heaped tablespoon of hummus
- A milky drink (e.g. milk, soya milk, latte or cappuccino) and a piece of fruit.
- A few oatcakes and a heaped tablespoon of hummus
- A slice of toast or two crispbreads with a slice of cheese
- A porridge scone (you can find a recipe for this in the second half of this book)
- A few vegetable mini frittatas (you can find a recipe for this in the second half of this book)
- A few dates with peanut butter

Plant-Based Food + High-Protein Food

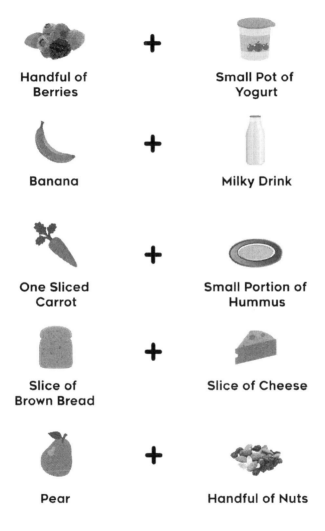

Handful of Berries + **Small Pot of Yogurt**

Banana + **Milky Drink**

One Sliced Carrot + **Small Portion of Hummus**

Slice of Brown Bread + **Slice of Cheese**

Pear + **Handful of Nuts**

Uncontrolled snacking:

There are a number of reasons why snacking can feel uncontrolled or distressing. For example, this can be triggered by extreme hunger, a lack of routine with your diet, emotional discomfort or feeling psychologically restricted and craving foods which you have placed 'off-limits'. I have listed common types of hunger below, as well as some strategies for addressing these.

Identifying your hunger type (these can also overlap):

- Physical hunger: This appears gradually when you have not eaten for a few hours, or if you have not been eating enough overall. You may feel low in energy, irritable, disoriented and have a gnawing empty feeling in your stomach.
- Taste hunger: This occurs when you have a specific food craving which is satisfied by eating a small to moderate portion of that food. It may be that you have not eaten a certain food in a while, or your diet may have become too repetitive.
- Emotional hunger: This type of hunger usually appears suddenly, without the signs of physical hunger being present. Emotional hunger is often associated with feeling sad, angry, frustrated, stressed, bored or tired.

Helpful strategies for physical hunger:

Try to eat every two to three hours by having three balanced meals and two to three balanced snacks every day (as outlined in this Chapter and Chapter 4). Make sure that you are eating enough to feel at least 70% full at mealtimes (where 0% is feeling ravenous and 100% is feeling uncomfortably stuffed). If you have increased your physical activity levels you may need to eat more or to adapt your nutritional intake to suit your training — if you are very active you may benefit from working with a Sports Nutritionist or Dietitian.

Helpful strategies for taste hunger:

Think about what textures or flavours your diet is missing and try to include a bigger variety of these in your meals and snacks. You may also need to work on slowly reintroducing foods that feel 'off limits' one at a time (i.e. foods you feel guilty or out of control around). Once you feel less anxious about reintroducing one food, you can move on to slowly reintroducing another food.

Helpful strategies for emotional hunger:

Reflecting on your feelings (by speaking to a loved one or journaling), practising mindfulness, relaxation techniques such as meditation and yoga, or working on acceptance skills and problem-solving in order to soothe your emotions. If this is persistent or challenging, you may benefit from support from a Psychologist or Therapist.

In some cases, feeling uncontrolled around food can be related to disordered eating. The following assessment was devised in collaboration with Dr Jake Linardon (PhD) — founder of breakbingeeating.com, Research Fellow and Psychology Lecturer at Deakin University in Melbourne, Australia.

Please answer yes or no to the following questions in relation to your eating experiences over the past month (i.e. 28 days):

1. In the past 28 days, have you eaten an unusually large amount of food in a short period of time, given the circumstances?
2. If you have eaten an unusually large amount of food, did you experience a sense of loss of control during this eating episode?
3. Are your judgments of self-worth (i.e. how you value yourself as a person) largely based on how much you weigh or how you look?
4. Does your eating make you feel extremely guilty, embarrassed or distressed?
5. Does this ever lead to purging (i.e. vomiting, use of laxatives or excessive exercise)?

If you answered yes to any of these questions I encourage you to speak to your doctor, and you may also benefit from seeking support from a Dietitian and a Therapist.

Chapter 6

Being a Food Realist

The final message I want to leave you with is the importance of a flexible approach and a balanced mindset when it comes to eating well. A realist can look at things logically, and deal with situations in a practical way. This is a really helpful approach to take when it comes to eating well. On the opposite end of the spectrum is the food perfectionist, who aims for an unrealistically flawless diet, obsesses over small details and is often hard on themselves.

The 'Perfect Diet' Illusion

Much of the anxiety related to trying to eat well is related to the pursuit of a 'perfect diet'. Striving for perfection in this way can lead to stress or avoidance of social occasions. This can also trigger an 'all or nothing' mindset, which can lead to cycles of yo-yo dieting or an unhealthy obsession with healthy eating (which has the potential to develop into an eating disorder). These behaviours are much worse for health and wellbeing as compared with the occasional takeaway or slice of cake.

A much healthier approach is to recognise that there is no such thing as one 'perfect diet' that suits us all 100% of the time, and that no specific foods are simply 'good or bad'. The bigger picture of what you eat most of the time, over the course of many years, impacts long-term health. So having an occasional chocolate bar doesn't unbalance the rest of your diet. Food also plays a much bigger role than simply providing nutrients — after all, enjoying tasty food is one of life's pleasures!

Adopting a flexible approach also makes eating well more realistic in the long term, as it reduces feelings of guilt when 'sometimes foods' are consumed, and breaks the cycle of feeling 'on or off the wagon'.

Another helpful approach to eating well is to focus on positive food additions, like adding more plants or oily fish to your diet, rather than focusing on cutting back and restricting your food intake.

Focusing on how you eat can also be useful. This can involve trying to eat more slowly and mindfully in order to really appreciate your food. Mindful eating can also help us to pay attention and respond to our feelings of hunger and fullness.

Processed Food Fear

Another common form of food perfectionism is feeling the need to cook all of your meals from scratch in order to have a healthy diet. When you have the time and motivation to cook from scratch this can be a great thing to do, but it isn't necessary all of the time.

This fear of processed foods is understandable, as they get a very bad rap. Although processed food can be high in salt, sugar or fat there are plenty of healthy processed foods available (as outlined in Chapters 2 and 3). Embracing options like tinned beans, wholegrain bread, frozen fruit and vegetables (etc.) makes it more realistic to whip up quick and balanced meals. So I encourage you to break free from meal preparation perfectionism, especially if you have a busy life.

If you are concerned that a specific processed food product may be unhealthy, then you can check the nutrition information on the label as outlined in Chapter 2.

As I have discussed throughout this book, flexibility is a vital part of a healthy relationship with food. So it is fine to occasionally consume processed foods which are higher in saturated fat, salt and sugar. But in the long term, we usually feel best when we consume these 'sometimes foods' less often and in smaller amounts than 'everyday foods' like fruit, vegetables, wholegrains, plant-based oils, nuts, seeds, meat and dairy (or vegan alternatives).

Ditch Fad Diets

Learning to spot nutritional nonsense is a liberating skill. This also saves you from wasting your precious time and money on pointless diets and supplements.

Here is my three-step approach for recognising nutritional nonsense:

Step 1: Is the person spreading the message qualified to understand nutrition science?

If they have a university-level degree in dietetics or nutrition they are more likely to be a reliable source of nutrition information, but of course, this depends on the individual and the message they are spreading. If not, then be cautious of their advice and perhaps seek clarification or support from a qualified nutrition professional.

Step 2: Watch out for nutritional red flags!

Look out for advice that seems to be unscientific, unhealthy or too good to be true.

Examples of nutritional red flags include:
- Very restrictive diets
- Dramatic weight-loss claims
- Promoting foods which 'detox' or 'cleanse the body' (this is nonsense!)
- So-called 'superfoods'
- Encouraging very high doses of supplements
- Diets that encourage non-foods like cotton wool, charcoal or clay (yes these diets exist!)
- Promoting non-medical food intolerance tests like IgG tests, kinesiology tests, hair tests and saliva tests[27]

Step 3: Does the claim appear to be backed by solid evidence?

This is the most important consideration, but also the most difficult to assess as nutrition studies are complicated to understand. This involves looking at whether there are any good quality studies to back up the claim.

Important factors to consider include:
- The type of study
- Whether it was peer-reviewed (i.e. reviewed by other experts in that area before being published)
- The size of the study
- How it was designed
- The results
- The limitations
- The overall body of evidence in this area

For those who don't have a background in nutrition science, it can be best to ask the opinion of a qualified nutrition professional. There are also some useful resources which examine nutrition headlines, including the Behind the Headlines website from the NHS. I also analyse the latest nutrition news stories in my monthly Dietetically Speaking newsletter.

The Bigger Picture of Health

Although nutrition has an important impact on health, we also need to acknowledge that this is just one factor involved in the bigger picture of overall health.

There are things which we can't change when it comes to our health, including genetics, age and sex. Socioeconomic factors also play a big role, such as our income, occupation, education and living situation. It is important not to overlook the significant impact these factors have on our lives and those around us.

Where possible, some of the most important health behaviours to focus on include:

- Nutrition — as discussed throughout this book.
- Regular movement — the minimum recommended activity level is 150 minutes per week of moderate-intensity activity (such as walking or cycling), plus strengthening exercise on at least two days per week (such as weight lifting, pilates or yoga).[28]
- Relaxation and stress management — different approaches work for different people, such as meditation, exercising, calling a friend, watching TV, drawing, listening to music or playing a game. It is worth making a list of activities which you find relaxing so that you start to build your own 'stress management toolkit'.
- Aiming for seven to nine hours of good quality sleep per night — there is more evidence emerging that regularly sleeping badly increases the risk of heart disease, diabetes and early death.[29]
- Limiting alcohol intake to 14 units per week — consuming too much alcohol is linked with a higher risk of: injuries, liver disease, heart disease, pancreatitis, sleep issues, mental health issues and certain types of cancer (especially breast, mouth and throat cancer).[16,30] One unit of alcohol is

approximately half a pint of 4% beer, half a medium glass of 13% wine or 25ml of spirits.[16] We should also have at least two alcohol-free days each week.[16]

- Regularly socialising — this has been shown to have benefits for mental health, immunity and overall wellbeing.[19-21]
- Not smoking, or seeking support to quit if you do smoke — smoking has a detrimental effect on lung, heart, brain, bone, skin and reproductive health.[31] It also significantly increases the risk of lung, stomach, mouth and throat cancer.
- Attending medical appointments, including check-ups and screening appointments.
- Good hand hygiene in order to reduce the risk of catching infections.

Zooming out and looking at the bigger picture of health highlights that it is counterproductive to aim for perfection in terms of nutrition, at the expense of other healthy lifestyle factors. The best thing we can do is to aim for overall balance in our lifestyle, most of the time. Of course, it is also important to embrace some flexibility with other lifestyle factors. For example, there will be some days where you need to prioritise rest above exercising or socialising.

Give Yourself a Break

There is no point in putting an unrealistic amount of pressure on yourself to eat 'perfectly' 100% of the time, as this usually leads to feelings of guilt and shame when you inevitably can't achieve this. As discussed above, the idea that there is 'one perfect diet' is a myth, and striving to achieve this may lead to a disordered relationship with food.

So I strongly encourage you to give yourself a break, treat yourself kindly and aim for 'good enough' rather than perfection. From my experience of working with clients, this approach leads to a much healthier relationship with food, and long-term improvements in diet quality which are easier to maintain.

This 'good enough' mindset can also be really helpful at times which are particularly stressful, or when it is simply unrealistic to prioritise healthy eating. At these times, it is important not to beat yourself up, as all you can do is your best. This may mean occasional short periods where your diet is less balanced than usual, it is important to be compassionate to yourself at these difficult times.

If you start to feel lost or confused about how to eat well, remember that your meals don't need to be fancy or extravagant. You can bring it back to basics and aim to base most of your meals on fruit or vegetables, carbohydrates, high-protein foods and a source of healthy fats — as outlined in Chapter 4. You can also create a tasty and balanced meal in a matter of minutes, using only a few ingredients — as you can see from many of the meal ideas I have included at the end of this book.

So I urge you to try the balanced and flexible path of the food realist, rather than the obsessive, stressful and unsustainable path of the food perfectionis

50 Quick and Balanced Meal Ideas

Understanding how to create a balanced meal is one thing, whereas putting this into practice can be an entirely different matter. So this section of the book includes 50 different meal ideas which are designed to be nutritious, convenient and of course, tasty!

Standard portion sizes for adults are used in the following recipes, so you may need to adapt these to suit your needs. For example, if you are very active or have a bigger build you may need to increase the portion sizes. The recipes can also be scaled up to feed more people, or for cooking in bulk and freezing extra portions. Options 43 to 50 work well for bulk cooking.

Ordinary dairy is used in these recipes, but vegans can replace this with a nutritious plant-based alternative, such as calcium-fortified soya milk or yogurt. You can also swap this for low-fat dairy if you prefer — although whole milk and ordinary plain yogurt are not high in fat or calories to begin with. Vegetarian or vegan alternatives (like tofu, tempeh, seitan, chickpeas, beans and lentils) can also be used as replacements in meals which contain meat, chicken or fish. Or vice versa, animal protein can be added to the vegetarian dishes included in this section.

In order to make these recipes as practical as possible, I have opted for a lot of convenient ingredients such as frozen fruit and vegetables. These can be replaced with fresh versions depending on your taste preferences, the ingredients you already have in the house and the amount of time you have available for meal preparation.

Please note: The nutritional content of these meal ideas has been calculated using Nutritics nutrition analysis software. This is always an estimation and these values may vary depending on the specific brands you use and how closely the recipe is followed.

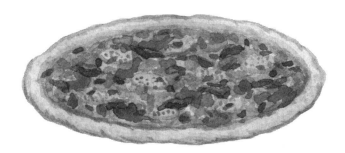

Breakfast Options:

Setting yourself up for the day with a nutritious breakfast is a great habit to get into. Options 1-8 can be eaten on the go if you don't have time for breakfast before you leave the house in the morning.

1. Apple and cinnamon overnight oats

Serves 1

Ingredients:
- ½ cup (40g) of oats
- 1 cup (200ml) of milk
- 1 grated apple
- 1 teaspoon of cinnamon
- 1 tablespoon of almond or peanut butter

Method:
1. Combine all of the ingredients in a tub or jar.
2. Store in the fridge overnight with the lid on, to be eaten cold the next morning.

Nutrition Information:

Kcal	Pro.	Fat	Sat. fat	Carb	Fibre	Added Sugar	Salt
480	17g	22g	7g	64g	8g	0g	0g

2. Vanilla berry overnight oats

Serves 1

Ingredients:
- ½ cup (40g) of oats
- ½ cup (100ml) of milk
- 2 tablespoons (100g) of natural yogurt
- 1 handful (30g) of flaked almonds
- 2 handfuls (80g) of berries
- ½ teaspoon of vanilla essence
- 1 tablespoon of chia seeds

Method:
1. Combine all of the ingredients in a tub or jar.
2. Store in the fridge overnight with the lid on, to be eaten cold the next morning.

Nutrition Information:

Kcal	Pro.	Fat	Sat. fat	Carb	Fibre	Added Sugar	Salt
530	22g	29g	7g	59g	14g	0g	0.3g

3. Carrot cake overnight oats

Serves 1

Ingredients:

- ½ cup (40g) of oats
- 1 cup (200ml) of milk
- 2 tablespoons of Greek yogurt
- ½ a medium carrot (grated)
- 1 tablespoon of chopped walnuts
- 1 heaped of tablespoon raisins
- 1 teaspoon of cinnamon
- ½ teaspoon of vanilla essence

Method:

1. Combine all of the ingredients in a tub or jar.
2. Store in the fridge overnight with the lid on, to be eaten cold the next morning.

Nutrition Information:

Kcal	Pro.	Fat	Sat. fat	Carb	Fibre	Added Sugar	Salt
540	20g	26g	13g	62g	6g	0g	0.5g

4. Tropical smoothie

Serves 1

Ingredients:
- 1 glass (200ml) of milk
- 3 tablespoons of yogurt
- ½ cup (40g) of oats
- 2 handfuls of frozen tropical fruit (pineapple, mango, etc.)
- 2 tablespoons of chia seeds
- 2 ice cubes

Method:
1. Blend all of the ingredients together until smooth — you can add some extra water or milk if you prefer a thinner consistency.
2. Serve in a glass or flask. This can also be made the night before and stored in the fridge.

Nutrition Information:

Kcal	Pro.	Fat	Sat. fat	Carb	Fibre	Added Sugar	Salt
490	23g	21g	8g	64g	11g	0g	0.5g

5. Berry smoothie

Serves 1

Ingredients:
- 1 glass (200ml) of milk
- ¼ cup (20g) of oats
- 1 tablespoon of Greek yogurt
- 1 banana
- 1 large handful of frozen berries
- 1 heaped tablespoon of nut butter
- 1 teaspoon of honey
- 2 ice cubes

Method:
1. Blend all of the ingredients together until smooth — you can add some extra water or milk if you prefer a thinner consistency.
2. Serve in a glass or flask. This can also be made the night before and stored in the fridge.

Nutrition Information:

Kcal	Pro.	Fat	Sat. fat	Carb	Fibre	Added Sugar	Salt
550	19g	28g	11g	61g	6g	0g	0.5g

6. Yogurt with granola

Serves 1

Ingredients:
- 3 tablespoons (150g) of Greek yogurt
- ½ a cup (50g) of granola (look for a version that doesn't have too much added sugar on the label — as outlined in the 'reading food labels' section of Chapter 2)
- 1 banana
- 1 handful of berries

Method:
1. Place the yogurt and granola in a bowl.
2. Top with berries and chopped banana and enjoy!

Nutrition Information:

Kcal	Pro.	Fat	Sat. fat	Carb	Fibre	Added Sugar	Salt
480	21g	25g	11g	51g	8g	4g	0.3g

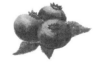

7. Porridge scones

Serves 4

Ingredients:
- 1 tub (450ml) of yogurt
- 350g of oats

To serve:
- 1 tablespoon of peanut butter per person
- 2 handfuls of fruit (any type you like!) per person

Method:
1. Preheat the oven to 180°C.
2. Combine the yogurt and oats in a mixing bowl.
3. Portion this mixture into a greased muffin tray and bake for about 30 minutes, until the scones are golden in colour and fully cooked in the middle.
4. Serve with peanut butter and around two handfuls of fruit per person — sliced banana, sliced pear or berries work well (this can be prepared in advance, and eaten cold).

Nutrition Information (per serving):

Kcal	Pro.	Fat	Sat. fat	Carb	Fibre	Added Sugar	Salt
540	20g	19g	5g	81g	9g	0g	0.4g

8. Mini vegetable frittatas

Serves 4

This is a great recipe to prepare in advance as it can be consumed cold or reheated in the microwave to save time in the morning. These are also a handy snack, and last 3-5 days in the fridge and 2-3 months in the freezer.

Ingredients:
- 2 cups (300g) of mixed vegetables (you can use leftover cooked vegetables, fresh chopped vegetables or frozen mixed vegetables)
- 1 cup (100g) of grated cheese
- 6 large eggs
- Black pepper to taste
- 2 slices of wholegrain toast per person
- 2 tablespoons of guacamole or 1 tablespoon of cream cheese per person

Method:
1. Preheat the oven to 200°C and grease a muffin tray.
2. If using frozen mixed vegetables, defrost in a pan or the microwave for three to four minutes. If using fresh chopped vegetables, steam or fry these until fully cooked.
3. Portion out the mixed vegetables and grated cheese into the muffin tray.
4. Whisk the eggs and add black pepper to taste, then pour this over the vegetables and cheese.

5. Bake for about 20 minutes, until the egg mixture has fully cooked through.
6. Divide these into four servings (usually 3-4 frittatas per person depending on the size of your muffin tray) and serve with two slices of wholegrain toast topped with guacamole or cream cheese.

Nutrition Information (per serving):

Kcal	Pro.	Fat	Sat. fat	Carb	Fibre	Added Sugar	Salt
440	28g	21g	9g	41g	7g	0g	1.5g

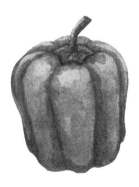

9. Wheat biscuit cereal with milk

Serves 1

Ingredients:
- 2 wheat biscuits (such as Weetabix or Wheat Bisks)
- 1 glass (200ml) of milk
- 2 handfuls of fruit
- 2 tablespoons of mixed seeds

Method:
1. Place the wheat biscuits and milk in a bowl.
2. Top with the fruit and mixed seeds — simple but effective!

Nutrition Information:

Kcal	Pro.	Fat	Sat. fat	Carb	Fibre	Added Sugar	Salt
460	18g	18g	6g	65g	7g	0g	0.6g

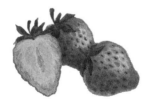

10. Banana and peanut butter porridge

Serves 1

Ingredients:
- 40g (½ cup) of oats
- 1 glass (200ml) of milk
- 1 banana
- 1 handful of berries
- 1 tablespoon of peanut butter

Method:
1. Combine the oats, milk and peanut butter in a small bowl and heat on full power in the microwave for about 90 seconds.
2. Then stir and microwave again for roughly 60 seconds (you may need to repeat this step a few times so that it thickens to your favourite porridge consistency).
3. Top with chopped banana and a handful of berries.

Nutrition Information:

Kcal	Pro.	Fat	Sat. fat	Carb	Fibre	Added Sugar	Salt
480	17g	20g	7g	65g	6g	0g	0.4g

11. Chocolate berry porridge

Serves 1

Ingredients:
- 40g (½ cup) of oats
- 1 glass (200ml) of milk
- 2 tablespoons of mixed nuts
- 2 handfuls of berries
- 1 teaspoon of cocoa powder (or 1 square of chocolate)

Method:
1. Combine the oats, milk and cocoa in a small bowl and heat on full power in the microwave for about 90 seconds.
2. Then stir and microwave again for roughly 60 seconds (you may need to repeat this step a few times so that it thickens to your favourite porridge consistency).
3. Top with the two handfuls of berries and two tablespoons of mixed nuts.

Nutrition Information:

Kcal	Pro.	Fat	Sat. fat	Carb	Fibre	Added Sugar	Salt
470	19g	25g	8g	48g	7g	0g	0.2g

12. Avocado toast with eggs

Serves 1

Ingredients:

- 2 slices of wholegrain bread
- ½ a medium avocado
- 2 poached eggs
- 1 handful of spinach
- 1 handful of cherry tomatoes
- Lemon juice and black pepper

Method:

1. Toast the bread and top this with sliced avocado.
2. Add a squirt of lemon juice on top of the avocado.
3. While poaching the eggs, wash the spinach and cherry tomatoes — this can be placed on top of the avocado or served on the side.
4. Once the eggs are poached to your liking (a runny yolk usually takes about three minutes), place these on top of the avocado toast and season with black pepper to taste.

Nutrition Information:

Kcal	Pro.	Fat	Sat. fat	Carb	Fibre	Added Sugar	Salt
520	24g	33g	8g	42g	10g	0g	1.1g

13. French toast

Serves 1

Ingredients:
- 2 slices of wholegrain bread
- 1 large egg
- 1 tablespoon of peanut or almond butter
- 1 small pot (½ cup or 125g) of yogurt
- 2 handfuls of berries
- 1 teaspoon of olive spread (or butter)

Method:
1. Crack the egg in a bowl, then whisk this using a fork or whisk.
2. Soak each side of the bread in the whisked egg.
3. Heat a teaspoon of spread (or butter) in a non-stick pan over a medium heat for about one minute. Then add the slices of eggy bread and fry for two to three minutes on each side, until they turn golden in colour.
4. Spread the nut butter on the French toast, then top this with the yogurt and berries.

Nutrition Information:

Kcal	Pro.	Fat	Sat. fat	Carb	Fibre	Added Sugar	Salt
530	28g	26g	8g	54g	8g	0g	1.4g

Breakfast Options

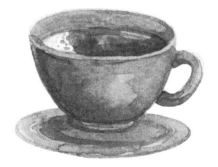

14. Banana pancakes

Serves 1

Ingredients:
- 1 banana
- 1 egg
- ½ cup (40g) of oats
- 1 tablespoon of nut butter
- 1 handful of fruit
- 125g pot of yogurt
- 1 teaspoon of olive or rapeseed oil

Method:
1. Blend the banana, egg and oats — or alternatively mash the egg and banana together using a fork, and then mix in the oats.
2. Heat the oil in a non-stick pan over a low to medium heat, then pour two to three ladles of the pancake mix into the pan (to make two to three separate mini pancakes).
3. Cook on each side for a few minutes until they are fully cooked and golden on each side.
4. Repeat until you have used up all of the batter.
5. Once cooked, spread the nut butter on the pancakes and top with yogurt and a handful of chopped fruit of your choice.

Nutrition Information:

Kcal	Pro.	Fat	Sat. fat	Carb	Fibre	Added Sugar	Salt
530	24g	21g	7g	68g	6g	0g	0.6g

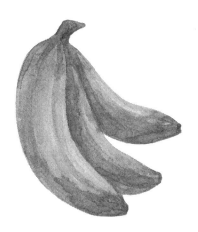

15. Vegetable omelette

Serves 1

Ingredients:
- 2 eggs
- 100ml of milk
- 30g (1 small handful) of grated cheese
- 1 medium pepper
- 1 handful of mushrooms
- 1 handful of spinach
- 1 teaspoon of vegetable oil
- 1-2 pressed garlic cloves (or 1 teaspoon of garlic purée)
- Black pepper
- 1 medium potato

Method:
1. Chop the potato into cubes, slice the peppers and mushrooms.
2. Steam the cubed potato in the microwave until this begins to soften (this usually takes at least five minutes).
3. Meanwhile, fry the peppers and garlic in a non-stick pan over a medium heat for three to four minutes in the vegetable oil. Then add the chopped mushrooms and fry for a further two to three minutes until the vegetables start to soften.

4. Add the potato to the pan and cook for three to four minutes until the potato and vegetables are fully cooked (add another drop of oil if the potato starts to stick to the pan).
5. Whisk the eggs and milk together, and add black pepper to taste.
6. Wash the spinach and add this to the pan — cook for about one minute until it wilts.
7. Pour the egg mix over the vegetables, and sprinkle the grated cheese on top.
8. Cook for two to three minutes, then place the pan under a medium grill to cook the top of the omelette and melt the cheese.

Nutrition Information:

Kcal	Pro.	Fat	Sat. fat	Carb	Fibre	Added Sugar	Salt
540	30g	29g	12g	42g	4g	1g	1.7g

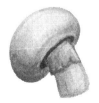

Lunch Options:

16. Hummus and vegetable wrap

Serves 1

Ingredients:

- 1 wholegrain wrap
- 2 tablespoons of hummus
- 1 slice of cheese
- 1 cup of frozen mixed Mediterranean vegetables (or fresh chopped peppers, courgette, aubergine, etc.)

Method:

1. If you are using a frozen vegetable mix, heat this in a pan until fully cooked. Otherwise prepare a batch of roasted vegetables using fresh peppers, courgette and aubergine — then add a few tablespoons of this to the wrap.
2. Spread the hummus on the wrap, add the cheese and vegetables and roll it up.

Nutrition Information:

Kcal	Pro.	Fat	Sat. fat	Carb	Fibre	Added Sugar	Salt
510	20g	29g	7g	51g	9g	2g	2g

17. Tuna salad sandwich

Serves 1

Ingredients:
- 2 slices of wholegrain bread
- 145g tin of tuna
- A few slices of cucumber
- 1 tablespoon of mayonnaise
- 2 tablespoons of sweetcorn
- 1 teaspoon of olive spread (or butter if you prefer)

Method:
1. Drain the tin of tuna and add to a bowl with the mayonnaise and sweetcorn. Then mix these ingredients together.
2. Butter the bread, place the sliced cucumber on this and then add the tuna mixture.
3. Slice the sandwich and enjoy!

Nutrition Information:

Kcal	Pro.	Fat	Sat. fat	Carb	Fibre	Added Sugar	Salt
530	40g	24g	2.5g	46g	8g	0g	1.3g

18. Chicken pesto pitta

Serves 1

Ingredients:

- 1 wholegrain pitta
- 1 cooked chicken fillet
- 1 tablespoon of red pesto
- ½ a red pepper
- 1 handful of spinach

Method:

1. Chop the chicken and pepper, wash and dry the spinach and slice the pitta in half.
2. Spread the pesto in the pitta then fill this with the chicken and vegetables.

Nutrition Information:

Kcal	Pro.	Fat	Sat. fat	Carb	Fibre	Added Sugar	Salt
450	47g	11g	2g	47g	7g	0g	1.2g

Lunch Options

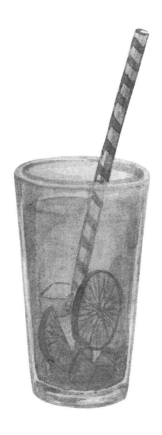

19. Mexican wrap

Serves 1

Ingredients:
- 1 wholegrain wrap
- 1 medium tomato
- 1 handful of spinach
- 1 tablespoon of natural yogurt
- 2 tablespoons of sweetcorn
- ½ a small avocado
- 100g of diced beef (vegetarians can swap this for 1 frozen bean burger)
- 1 teaspoon of chilli powder
- 1 teaspoon of vegetable or olive oil

Method:
1. Fry the beef in the oil and chilli powder until it has browned. If using the bean burger instead, cook this as per the instructions on the packet, then slice longways (this can be eaten hot or cold).
2. Slice the tomato and avocado, wash and dry the spinach.
3. Add the beef (or sliced bean burger) to the wrap, followed by the tomato, sweetcorn, avocado and spinach.
4. Top with one tablespoon of natural yogurt (or sour cream).

Nutrition Information:

Kcal	Pro.	Fat	Sat. fat	Carb	Fibre	Added Sugar	Salt
610	34g	31g	8g	57g	9g	2g	1.2g

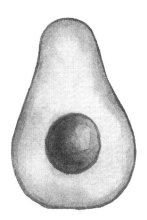

20. Lentil and vegetable soup

Serves 4

This soup can be made in advance and it also freezes very well, so it is a good recipe for batch meal preparation. To balance this meal, the soup is served with a cheese sandwich in this example — feel free to swap this for another type of sandwich which includes a high protein filling e.g. chicken, turkey, egg, etc.

Ingredients:
- 2 medium onions
- 2-3 garlic cloves
- 1 tablespoon of olive or rapeseed oil
- Whichever mixed vegetables you fancy, for example: 3 carrots, 1 courgette, 2 sticks of celery, ½ a packet of mushrooms, 1 red pepper
- 1 low-salt vegetable stock cube
- 1 tin of chopped tomatoes
- 300g of red split lentils
- 2 slices of wholegrain bread and a 25g slice of cheese per person
- Olive spread (or butter)

Method:

1. Dice the onion and garlic (or use a garlic press if you prefer).
2. Fry the onion and garlic in one to two tablespoons of oil over a medium heat until the onion starts to become translucent.
3. Chop the rest of your vegetables, then sauté until they begin to soften.
4. Add the lentils and cover with 450ml of vegetable stock.
5. Stir in the tin of tomatoes.
6. Simmer until the lentils are cooked — you may need to add some extra boiling water if you prefer a thinner consistency (you can also add extra herbs and spices to taste).
7. While the soup is cooking, make a cheese sandwich or cheese toastie to serve with the soup. If you have prepared the soup in advance, simply reheat this while you are making your sandwich.

Nutrition Information (per serving):

Kcal	Pro.	Fat	Sat. fat	Carb	Fibre	Added Sugar	Salt
470	21g	19g	6g	67g	13g	0g	1.3g

21. Mexican bean soup

Serves 2

Ingredients:
- 400g tin of taco beans
- 400g tin of chopped tomatoes
- 1 handful of frozen peppers (or 1 fresh pepper, chopped)
- 1 handful of frozen onions (or 1 small fresh onion, chopped)
- 200g tin of sweetcorn
- 1 teaspoon of dried coriander
- 1 teaspoon of dried cumin
- 2 teaspoons of chilli powder (or more if you like it spicy)
- 1 wholegrain pitta bread per person
- 2 tablespoons of guacamole per person

Method:
1. Combine the taco beans, tinned tomatoes, peppers, onions, sweetcorn and spices in a pan (you can add a second tin of tomatoes or some water if you like your soup to be a thinner consistency). If using fresh onion and pepper, sauté these in a pan until they begin to soften before adding the other ingredients.
2. Bring this to the boil and simmer, stirring as needed, until all of the vegetables are cooked.
3. Serve this with a wholegrain pitta filled with guacamole (or top the soup with the guacamole).

Nutrition Information (per serving):

Kcal	Pro.	Fat	Sat. fat	Carb	Fibre	Added Sugar	Salt
480	10g	10g	2.5g	95g	19g	0g	1g

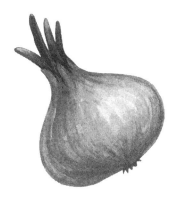

22. Heart-healthy chowder

Serves 2

Ingredients:
- 500ml of milk
- 320g of fish pie mix (or you can make your own mix using white fish, salmon and prawns)
- 1 medium onion
- 1 leek
- 1 large potato
- 1 clove of garlic
- 100g of frozen peas
- 1 teaspoon of vegetable oil
- 1 teaspoon of dried thyme
- 500ml of reduced-salt vegetable stock
- Black pepper to taste
- 1 handful of parsley
- 1 slice of brown bread per person

Method:
1. Put the fish pie mix in a large pan with the milk and stock, bring to the boil, then reduce the heat to simmer.
2. Dice the onion, leek and potato, and crush the garlic.
3. Sauté the onion, garlic, leek and vegetable oil on a medium heat for about five minutes (until they start to soften).
4. Add the potato and cook for a further two to three minutes.

5. Add the onion, leek and potato to the pan with the fish in it, along with the peas, thyme and black pepper. Simmer for 15 to 20 minutes until the fish and potato are fully cooked.

6. Garnish with chopped parsley and serve with a slice of brown bread per person.

Nutrition Information (per serving):

Kcal	Pro.	Fat	Sat. fat	Carb	Fibre	Added Sugar	Salt
670	43g	22g	8g	76g	12g	0g	2g

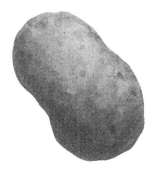

23. Minestrone soup

Serves 4

Ingredients:
- 400g tin of chopped tomatoes
- 120g of spaghetti snapped into small pieces (or you can use a small type of pasta, such as ditalini)
- 350g of frozen mixed peas and sweetcorn
- 1 medium onion or 1 cup (150g) of frozen onion
- 400g tin of cannellini beans
- 2 tablespoons of pesto
- 1 tablespoon of olive or vegetable oil
- 1 litre of reduced-salt vegetable stock (i.e. 2 stock cubes in 1 litre of boiling water)
- 4 small handfuls (80g) of grated cheese
- Serve with 1-2 slices wholegrain bread per person

Method:
1. Chop the onion then sauté this in a tablespoon of oil in a saucepan over a medium heat for two to three minutes (if using frozen chopped onions skip this step).
2. Add the stock, pesto, tinned tomatoes and pasta to the pan, then bring this to the boil and cook for about five minutes (until this starts to soften).
3. Add the peas, sweetcorn and cannellini beans to the pan and simmer for two to three minutes until all ingredients are cooked.
4. Serve with grated cheese, a drizzle of olive oil and a slice of wholegrain bread per person.

Nutrition Information (per serving):

Kcal	Pro.	Fat	Sat. fat	Carb	Fibre	Added Sugar	Salt
420	19g	14g	6g	62g	11g	0g	1.8g

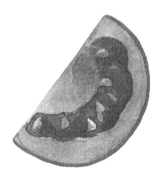

24. Middle Eastern salad

Serves 2

Ingredients:
- 400g tin of lentils
- 100g of dry couscous
- 2 tablespoons of hummus
- 2 tablespoons of olive oil
- The juice of half a lemon
- 2 handfuls of chopped cucumber
- 2 medium tomatoes
- 1 pepper

Method:
1. Add the couscous to a bowl, cover with boiling water and cover with a lid or plate. Leave this to stand for a few minutes — you may need to add more water if the couscous absorbs all of the water without fully softening.
2. Chop the tomato, cucumber and pepper. Once the couscous is fully cooked, stir in the chopped vegetables.
3. Drain and rinse the lentils before adding to the couscous, along with the olive oil and lemon juice.
4. Mix all of the ingredients together and serve with a tablespoon of hummus on the side.

Nutrition Information (per serving):

Kcal	Pro.	Fat	Sat. fat	Carb	Fibre	Added Sugar	Salt
610	27g	23g	3g	88g	15g	0g	0.5g

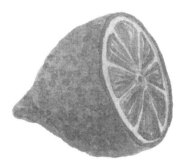

25. Falafel salad

Serves 2

Ingredients:

- 8 ready-made falafels
- 250g bag of microwave wholegrain rice and quinoa (or 100g of dried quinoa)
- 1 red pepper
- 1 pickled beetroot
- 2 handfuls of spinach
- 100g of feta (½ of a packet)
- 2 tablespoons of hummus
- Lemon juice
- Olive oil

Method:

1. If using dried quinoa and falafels which are not pre-cooked, cook these as per the instructions on the packet (otherwise skip this step).
2. Wash the spinach and chop the beetroot, pepper and feta.
3. Mix the quinoa, chopped vegetables and feta in a bowl with a drizzle of olive oil and a squirt of lemon juice. Divide the salad into two servings, add four falafels on top of the salad and a tablespoon of hummus on the side of each serving.

Nutrition Information (per serving):

Kcal	Pro.	Fat	Sat. fat	Carb	Fibre	Added Sugar	Salt
590	22g	27g	6g	82g	17g	2g	1.9g

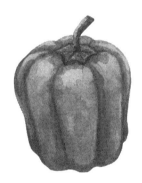

26. Pesto pasta salad

Serves 1

Ingredients:
- 60g of uncooked wholemeal pasta
- 1 small cooked chicken fillet
- 2 tablespoons of pesto
- 1 large handful of cherry tomatoes
- 1 large handful of spinach

Method:
1. Cook the pasta as per the instructions on the packet.
2. Chop the cooked chicken fillet into bite-sized pieces.
3. Once the pasta is cooked, combine all of the ingredients together in the pan — this can be eaten hot or cold.

Nutrition Information:

Kcal	Pro.	Fat	Sat. fat	Carb	Fibre	Added Sugar	Salt
550	41g	24g	4g	50g	8g	0g	1.8g

27. Tuna pasta salad

Serves 1

Ingredients:
- 60g of uncooked wholemeal pasta
- 1 small (80g) tin of tuna
- 1 tablespoon of mayonnaise
- 2 tablespoons of sweetcorn
- ½ a pepper
- 1 carrot

Method:
1. Cook the pasta as per the instructions on the packet.
2. While this is cooking, chop the pepper and grate the carrot.
3. Once the pasta is cooked, stir in the tuna, mayonnaise, sweetcorn, pepper and grated carrot — this can be eaten hot or cold.

Nutrition Information:

Kcal	Pro.	Fat	Sat. fat	Carb	Fibre	Added Sugar	Salt
560	35g	16g	2g	85g	14g	0g	1.7g

28. Prawn cocktail salad

Serves 1

Ingredients:

- 100g of cooked prawns
- 1 tablespoon of mayonnaise
- 1 tablespoon of ketchup
- ½ an avocado
- 1 handful of cherry tomatoes
- 1 spring onion
- Lemon juice
- 1 handful of lettuce
- 1 handful of spinach
- 1 small potato (roughly 100g)

Method:

1. Chop the potato into cubes and steam in the microwave until this is fully cooked (this usually takes at least 5 minutes). Leave this to cool.
2. Mix the prawns, mayonnaise and ketchup together.
3. Chop the avocado, cherry tomatoes and spring onion, and wash the lettuce.
4. Add the chopped vegetables, lettuce, cooled potatoes and a squirt of lemon juice to a bowl and mix these together.
5. Serve with the prawn mixture on top of the salad.

Nutrition Information:

Kcal	Pro.	Fat	Sat. fat	Carb	Fibre	Added Sugar	Salt
550	22g	36g	5g	42g	7g	7g	2.1g

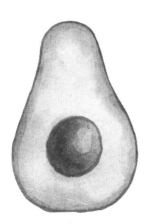

29. High-fibre salad

Serves 2

Ingredients:

- 250g microwave bag of cooked grains e.g. quinoa and bulgur wheat (or 100g of dried quinoa)
- 400g tin of chickpeas
- ½ a medium cucumber
- 1 red pepper
- 50g of cheddar cheese
- 2 handfuls of fresh or frozen pomegranate seeds
- 2 tablespoons of olive oil
- The juice of ½ a lemon
- Black pepper to taste
- 1 handful of coriander

Method:

1. If using dried quinoa, cook this as per the instructions on the packet (otherwise skip this step).
2. Chop the pepper, cucumber, coriander and cheese into bite-sized pieces.
3. If using frozen pomegranate seeds defrost these in the microwave.
4. Mix all ingredients together, or keep each food separate and serve like a Buddha bowl.

Nutrition Information (per serving):

Kcal	Pro.	Fat	Sat. fat	Carb	Fibre	Added Sugar	Salt
640	30g	23g	23g	101g	23g	0g	1.2g

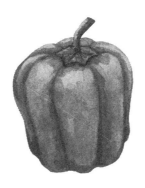

30. Greek bulgur wheat salad

Serves 4

Ingredients:
- 1 head of broccoli
- 200g of uncooked bulgur wheat (or 2 x 250g packets of pre-cooked bulgur wheat and quinoa)
- 2 handfuls of cherry tomatoes
- 400g tin of lentils
- 200g packet of feta
- 2 large handfuls of mixed nuts and raisins (80g)
- Lemon juice
- 2 tablespoons of olive oil
- 1 tablespoon of balsamic vinegar

Method:
1. Cook the bulgur wheat as per the instructions on the label (or if you are short on time use two 250g packets of pre-cooked bulgur wheat and quinoa instead).
2. Wash and chop the broccoli, then steam this for roughly five minutes until it has softened.
3. Chop the tomatoes and feta into bite-sized chunks.
4. Then mix the bulgur wheat, steamed broccoli, chopped tomato, chopped feta, drained tin of lentils, nuts, raisins, olive oil, balsamic vinegar and a squirt of lemon juice together in a bowl.

Nutrition Information (per serving):

Kcal	Pro.	Fat	Sat. fat	Carb	Fibre	Added Sugar	Salt
600	27g	25g	9g	78g	10g	0g	1.3g

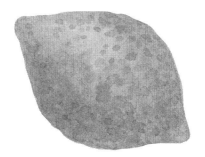

Dinner Options:

31. Creamy salmon pasta

Serves 2

Ingredients:

- 120g of uncooked wholemeal pasta
- 2 handfuls of frozen peas
- ½ a head of broccoli (or 2 large handfuls of frozen broccoli)
- 1 medium onion (or 1 large handful of frozen onion)
- 2 tablespoons of cream cheese
- 4 tablespoons of natural yogurt
- 100g smoked salmon
- 2 cloves of garlic (or 1 teaspoon of garlic purée)
- Black pepper to taste
- Lemon juice

Method:

1. Boil the pasta for five minutes. If there is a lot of excess water, drain some of this off so there is about half an inch (roughly 3cm) of water above the pasta.
2. Chop the onion, broccoli and smoked salmon into bite-sized pieces. Crush or finely chop the garlic.
3. Sauté the onion, garlic and broccoli over a medium heat with a small amount of oil for about three minutes, until these start to soften (if using frozen vegetables skip this step).

4. Add the onion, broccoli, salmon, peas, cream cheese, yogurt, pepper and a squirt of lemon juice to the pot with the pasta.
5. Bring to the boil, then simmer until the pasta and vegetables are fully cooked, stirring as needed.

Nutrition Information (per serving):

Kcal	Pro.	Fat	Sat. fat	Carb	Fibre	Added Sugar	Salt
590	35g	24g	12g	72g	13g	0g	2.9g

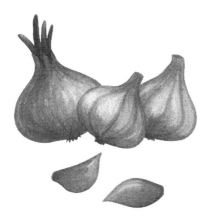

32. Wrap pizza

Serves 1

Ingredients:
- 2 tablespoons of tomato purée
- 1 wholegrain wrap
- 1 handful of grated mozzarella
- 1 spring onion
- 1 handful of mushrooms
- 1 handful of spinach
- 1 handful mixed leaves
- 1 medium tomato
- 1 teaspoon of olive oil

Method:
1. Chop the spring onion, slice the mushrooms, wash and dry the spinach.
2. Spread the tomato purée on the wrap, then sprinkle a handful of grated mozzarella on top of the wrap, followed by the toppings (spring onion, mushroom and spinach).
3. Grill this under a medium heat until the toppings are cooked.
4. Serve with a side salad of mixed leaves and chopped tomato with a drizzle of olive oil on top.

Nutrition Information:

Kcal	Pro.	Fat	Sat. fat	Carb	Fibre	Added Sugar	Salt
560	23g	26g	9g	73g	14g	4g	1.6g

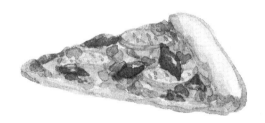

33. Baked potato with tuna

Serves 1

Ingredients:

- 1 medium potato
- 145g tin of tuna
- 1 tablespoon of mayonnaise
- ½ a red pepper
- 3 tablespoons of sweetcorn
- ½ a small avocado

Method:

1. Either bake the potato in the oven, or cook it in the microwave by pricking with a fork a few times then heating the potato on full power for four to five minutes, then turn the potato over, and microwave for a further four to five minutes.
2. Chop the pepper and mix this with the drained tin of tuna, mayonnaise and sweetcorn.
3. Once the potato is cooked, slice it in half and add the tuna mixture. Top with sliced avocado.

Alternative toppings include: bean chilli or beans and cheese.

Nutrition Information:

Kcal	Pro.	Fat	Sat. fat	Carb	Fibre	Added Sugar	Salt
540	38g	33g	5g	32g	8g	1g	1.1g

34. Fancy beans on toast

Serves 1

Ingredients:

- 2 slices of wholegrain bread
- 2 teaspoons of olive spread (or butter)
- 1 small (200g) tin of baked beans (or ½ of a ordinary 400g tin)
- 2 handfuls of mushrooms
- 1 small handful of grated cheese (20g)
- 1 tablespoon of mixed seeds

Method:

1. Chop and grill the mushrooms (or use frozen chopped mushrooms and heat these up in a pan).
2. Heat up the beans in the microwave, toast the bread and add spread.
3. Add the mushrooms and beans on top of the toast.
4. Top with grated cheese and mixed seeds.

Nutrition Information:

Kcal	Pro.	Fat	Sat. fat	Carb	Fibre	Added Sugar	Salt
550	26g	22g	7g	76g	16g	8g	2.5g

35. Five-minute mackerel risotto

Serves 2

Ingredients:
- 250g bag of pre-cooked microwave rice
- 1 handful of frozen peas
- 1 handful of frozen sliced peppers
- 2 tins (120g each) of chilli mackerel
- 2 heaped tablespoons of natural yogurt
- 100ml of milk
- Black pepper to taste

Method:
1. Combine all ingredients in a pan over a medium heat.
2. Heat this mixture until everything is cooked through, stirring as needed (this usually only takes about five minutes).

Nutrition Information (per serving):

Kcal	Pro.	Fat	Sat. fat	Carb	Fibre	Added Sugar	Salt
580	33g	21g	6g	69g	5g	0g	1.3g

Dinner Options

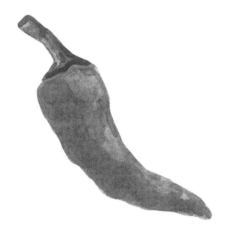

36. Chicken and vegetable fried rice

Serves 2

Ingredients:

- 1 large chicken breast (or 2 small chicken breasts)
- 1 tablespoon of olive or vegetable oil
- 6 handfuls of frozen stir-fry mix vegetables (or a variety of fresh vegetables, chopped)
- 250g bag of microwave rice (or 100g of dried rice)
- 1 egg
- 1 tablespoon of soy sauce
- 1 handful of mixed nuts

Method:

1. If using dried rice, cook this as per the instructions on the packet (skip this step if using a pouch of pre-cooked rice).
2. Chop the chicken breast, then fry this in a wok or pan with the vegetable oil and soy sauce.
3. When the chicken is cooked, add the frozen stir-fry mixed vegetables and cook for two to three minutes (if using fresh versions, you will need to stir-fry this for longer until the vegetables start to soften).
4. Then add the rice and cook for a further two minutes.
5. Add the nuts and crack the egg into the pan, then stir continuously until the rice is piping hot and the egg has been fully cooked.

Nutrition Information:

Kcal	Pro.	Fat	Sat. fat	Carb	Fibre	Added Sugar	Salt
580	42g	21g	3.5g	63g	9g	1g	2.2g

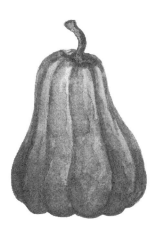

37. Courgette fritters with poached eggs

Serves 1

Ingredients:
- 1 large courgette
- 1 small carrot
- 1 handful of chopped spinach
- 3 eggs
- Nutmeg
- 1 spring onion
- 1 medium potato
- 1 tablespoon of olive or rapeseed oil

Method:
1. Grate the courgette and carrot, chop the spring onion, cube the potato and whisk one egg.
2. Mix the courgette and carrot with the chopped spinach, whisked egg, spring onion and a small sprinkle of grated nutmeg.
3. Make into patties and fry on each side.
4. Meanwhile, steam the potatoes in the microwave for about five minutes, then fry these in oil in a separate pan over a medium heat for a further five to ten minutes (until crisp and golden brown).
5. Poach the two remaining eggs while the patties and potatoes are frying.
6. To serve: top the fritters with the poached eggs and serve the fried potatoes on the side.

Nutrition Information:

Kcal	Pro.	Fat	Sat. fat	Carb	Fibre	Added Sugar	Salt
530	33g	28g	7g	44g	9g	0g	0.7g

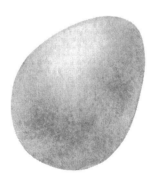

38. Greek omelette

Serves 1

Ingredients:

- 2 eggs
- 50g of feta cheese (¼ packet)
- 1 handful of mushrooms
- 1 handful of spinach
- 2 slices of wholegrain toast
- 1 tablespoon of olive spread or butter
- Nutmeg
- Olive oil

Method:

1. Heat a teaspoon of olive oil over a medium heat in a non-stick pan for about a minute, then add the mushrooms and fry for two to three minutes.
2. Add the spinach and cook for a further minute.
3. Whisk the eggs and add grated nutmeg to taste.
4. Chop the feta.
5. Add the egg mixture to the pan along with the feta.
6. Cook the underside of the omelette in the pan for three to four minutes, then transfer to the grill and cook the top of the omelette under a medium heat until the egg is cooked through.
7. Serve with two slices of wholegrain toast with spread or butter (alternatively you could have fried potatoes as a side).

Nutrition Information:

Kcal	Pro.	Fat	Sat. fat	Carb	Fibre	Added Sugar	Salt
490	24g	30g	11g	38g	7g	3g	2.4g

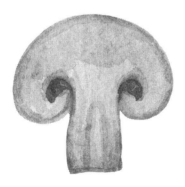

39. Lemon and basil fish

Serves 1

Ingredients:

- 1 medium fillet of white fish, such as cod or haddock
- 6 new potatoes
- 1 handful of broccoli
- 1 handful of cauliflower
- 1 medium carrot
- The juice of ½ a lemon
- 1 tablespoon of olive oil
- 1 small handful of fresh basil
- 1 clove of garlic

Method:

1. Preheat the oven to 200°C.
2. Chop the basil using kitchen scissors and crush the clove of garlic.
3. In a bowl, mix the basil, garlic, lemon juice and olive oil together.
4. Place the fish in tinfoil. Pour the lemon and basil mixture over the fish and close the tinfoil over the top (so the fish is wrapped loosely in a tin foil parcel). Place this in the oven for 10 to 15 minutes.
5. As the fish is baking, wash and chop the potatoes and vegetables.
6. Steam the potatoes for five minutes, then add the rest of the vegetables and steam for a further five minutes. You may need to repeat this step to ensure that the potatoes and vegetables are fully cooked.
7. Serve the fish, potatoes and vegetables together.

Nutrition Information:

Kcal	Pro.	Fat	Sat. fat	Carb	Fibre	Added Sugar	Salt
470	34g	15g	2.5g	52g	10g	0g	0.5g

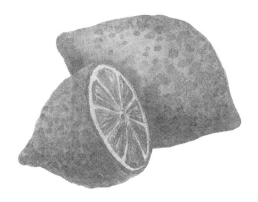

40. Simple beef stir-fry

Serves 4

Ingredients:

- 600g packet of frozen stir-fry vegetable mix (or a variety of chopped fresh vegetables)
- 2 tablespoons of olive or rapeseed oil
- 2 tablespoons of soy sauce
- 2 teaspoons of chilli powder
- 400g of diced beef steak (or swap this for 2 large chicken fillets or 1 block of pressed tofu)
- 50g of rice (uncooked weight) per person (or half of a 250g cooked microwave bag of rice per person)

Method:

1. Boil the rice as per the instructions on the packet.
2. Fry the diced beef steak (or chicken or tofu) in a wok or pan with the oil, soy sauce and chilli powder.
3. When the beef has browned, add the mixed vegetables and cook for two to three minutes (if using fresh chopped vegetables, you will need to stir-fry this for longer until the vegetables start to soften).
4. Serve with the rice, and enjoy!

Nutrition Information:

Kcal	Pro.	Fat	Sat. fat	Carb	Fibre	Added Sugar	Salt
520	30g	19g	3.5g	64g	8g	1g	2g

Dinner Options

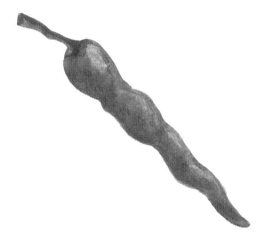

41. Chilli salmon stir-fry

Serves 1

Ingredients:
- 1 salmon fillet
- 1 tablespoon of olive or rapeseed oil
- Chilli flakes
- 3 handfuls of frozen vegetable stir-fry mix (or a variety of chopped fresh vegetables)
- 1 nest of wholegrain noodles
- 1 tablespoon of soy sauce

Method:
1. Preheat the oven to 200°C.
2. Place a fillet of salmon in tin foil, top with one teaspoon of olive oil and chilli flakes to taste, close the tin foil over the salmon (so the fish is wrapped loosely in a tin foil parcel) and bake for 10 to 15 minutes (or alternatively, heat up a ready-cooked chilli salmon fillet).
3. While the salmon is cooking, stir-fry the mixed vegetables in a wok with the soy sauce until the vegetables start to soften.
4. Boil a nest of wholegrain noodles as per the instructions on the packet, then mix the vegetables into the noodles.
5. Serve the chilli salmon on top of a bed of mixed noodles and vegetables.

Nutrition Information:

Kcal	Pro.	Fat	Sat. fat	Carb	Fibre	Added Sugar	Salt
540	30g	26g	4.5g	49g	5g	0g	1.1g

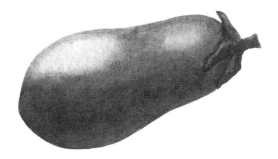

42. Chilli beef hash

Serves 4

Ingredients:

- 3 medium potatoes
- 500g of lean minced beef
- 2 cups (300g) of frozen peas
- 340g tin of sweetcorn
- 1 medium onion
- 1 teaspoon of chilli powder
- 1 teaspoon of paprika
- 1 teaspoon of cumin
- 1 tablespoon of olive or rapeseed oil

Method:

1. Chop the onion and dice the potatoes into small cubes.
2. Steam the potatoes in the microwave for about five minutes, then fry these in oil over a medium heat for a further five to ten minutes (until crisp and golden brown).
3. Meanwhile, sauté the onion in a small amount of oil for two to three minutes, then add the minced beef to this and cook until brown.
4. Add the peas, sweetcorn, fried potatoes and seasoning to the mince and cook for four to five minutes, stirring as needed, until all ingredients are cooked through.

Nutrition Information (per serving):

Kcal	Pro.	Fat	Sat. fat	Carb	Fibre	Added Sugar	Salt
500	26g	16g	3g	72g	11g	1g	1g

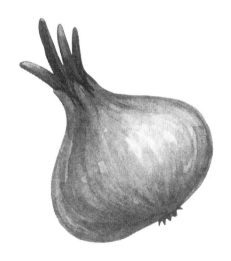

43. Chicken and chickpea curry

Serves 2

Ingredients:
- 2 chicken fillets (or a 280g block of pressed tofu)
- 400g tin of chickpeas
- 400g tin of chopped tomatoes
- 2 tablespoons of curry powder
- 1 teaspoon of dried coriander
- 1 teaspoon of cumin
- 4 tablespoons of natural yogurt
- 1 medium pepper (or 2 handfuls of frozen peppers)
- 1 medium onion (or 1 handful of frozen onions)
- 1 handful of mushrooms (fresh or frozen)
- 2-3 cloves of garlic (or 1-2 teaspoons of garlic purée)
- 100g of rice (uncooked weight) or a 250g bag of pre-cooked rice

Method:
1. Chop the chicken into bite-sized pieces, then fry in the oil and spices (curry powder, dried coriander and cumin) until fully cooked.
2. Meanwhile, finely chop the onion and garlic and chop the mushrooms and pepper into bite-sized pieces.
3. Add the onion and garlic to the pan and fry for one to two minutes.
4. Then add the peppers and fry for two to three minutes, followed by the mushrooms and fry for a further two to three minutes (if using frozen vegetables, add these all at the same time).

5. Boil the rice as per the instructions on the packet.
6. Add the tinned tomatoes, chickpeas and natural yogurt. Bring to the boil and simmer on a low heat for around 10 minutes, until all of the vegetables are cooked.

Nutrition Information (per serving):

Kcal	Pro.	Fat	Sat. fat	Carb	Fibre	Added Sugar	Salt
570	41g	9g	1.5g	79g	14g	3g	1.3g

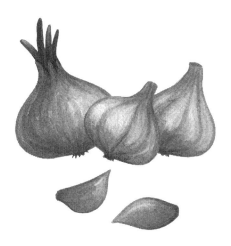

44. Lentil bolognese

Serves 2

Ingredients:
- 400g tin of lentils
- 400g tin of chopped tomatoes
- 1 tablespoon of tomato purée
- 2-3 cloves of garlic (or 1-2 teaspoons of garlic purée)
- 1 medium pepper (or 2 handfuls of frozen peppers)
- 1 medium onion (or 1 handful of frozen onions)
- 1 handful of mushrooms (fresh or frozen)
- 1 teaspoon of oregano
- 1 teaspoon of dried basil
- 120g of uncooked wholemeal pasta

Method:
1. Cook the pasta as per the instructions on the packet.
2. Dice the onion and garlic, then sauté in a pan over a medium heat for one to two minutes.
3. Chop the pepper and mushrooms, then add the chopped pepper to the pan and fry for two to three minutes, followed by the mushrooms for a further two to three minutes (if using frozen vegetables, add these all at the same time).
4. Add the tinned tomatoes, tomato purée, lentils, oregano and basil.
5. Bring this to the boil, then simmer gently for about 10 minutes.
6. Drain the pasta, and serve this with the lentil bolognese sauce. You can also add a sprinkle of cheddar cheese, parmesan cheese or nutritional yeast.

Nutrition Information (per serving):

Kcal	Pro.	Fat	Sat. fat	Carb	Fibre	Added Sugar	Salt
610	33g	10g	1.5g	119g	22g	8g	1.3g

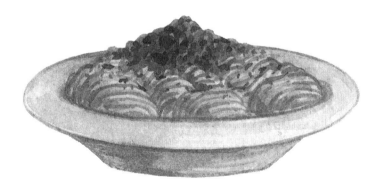

45. Lentil and butterbean stew

Serves 2

Ingredients:

- 400g tin of lentils
- 400g tin of butter beans
- 400g tin of chopped tomatoes
- 1 medium onion (or 1 handful of frozen chopped onion)
- Half a head of broccoli (or 1 handful of frozen broccoli)
- 1 reduced-salt vegetable stock cube
- 2-3 cloves of garlic (or 1-2 teaspoons of garlic purée)
- 2 teaspoons of chilli powder
- ½ a teaspoon of sugar
- Oregano and basil to taste
- 1 medium baked or microwaved potato per person
- 1 tablespoon of olive or rapeseed oil

Method:

1. Chop the onion and broccoli, crush the garlic.
2. Heat a tablespoon of oil in a saucepan over a medium heat, then add the onion and garlic and sauté for two to three minutes.
3. Add the lentils, butter beans, tin of tomatoes, vegetables, garlic, sugar, herbs and spices to the pan over a medium heat.
4. Dissolve the vegetable stock cube in a small amount of boiled water and add this to the pan. Bring to the boil and simmer for 10 to 15 minutes until all of the vegetables are cooked.

5. Serve with a baked or microwaved potato (you can find instructions for microwaving a potato in option 33. Baked potato with tuna).

Nutrition Information (per serving):

Kcal	Pro.	Fat	Sat. fat	Carb	Fibre	Added Sugar	Salt
540	37g	3.5g	0.5g	111g	21g	3g	0.9g

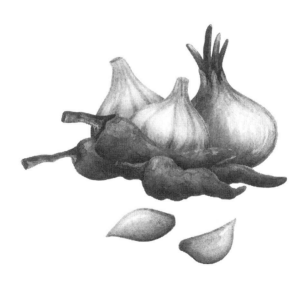

46. Bean chilli

Serves 3

Ingredients:
- 400g tin of taco beans
- 400g tin of kidney beans
- 400g tin of chopped tomatoes
- 1 medium pepper (or 2 handfuls of frozen peppers)
- 1 medium onion (or 1 handful of frozen onions)
- 100g of sweetcorn
- 2 teaspoons of chilli powder (you can add more, depending on how spicy you like it)
- 50g of rice (uncooked weight) per person (or half of a 250g cooked microwave bag of rice per person)

Method:
1. Dice the onion and garlic, then sauté in a pan over a medium heat for one to two minutes.
2. Chop the pepper, then add to the pan with the onion and garlic and fry for a further two to three minutes (if using frozen vegetables, add the onion and peppers to the pan at the same time).
3. Boil the rice as per the instructions on the packet.
4. Add the taco beans, kidney beans, tinned tomatoes, sweetcorn and chilli powder to the pan.
5. Bring to the boil and simmer for around 10 minutes until all of the vegetables are fully cooked.
6. Serve on a bed of rice.

Nutrition Information (per serving):

Kcal	Pro.	Fat	Sat. fat	Carb	Fibre	Added Sugar	Salt
440	25g	5g	1g	101g	23g	0g	0.5g

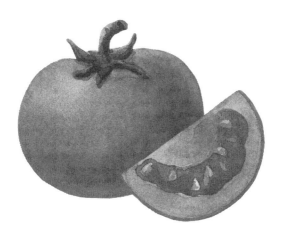

47. Quesadillas

Serves 1

Ingredients:
- 1 teaspoon of vegetable oil
- 2 wholemeal wraps
- 4-5 tablespoons of bean chilli (see recipe 46)
- 1 small handful (30g) of cheese
- 1 heaped tablespoon of guacamole

Method:
1. Heat a teaspoon of vegetable oil in a non-stick frying pan over a low to medium heat.
2. Add a wholemeal wrap to the pan, followed by four to five tablespoons of bean chilli on top of the wrap and spread this evenly using the back of a spoon.
3. Then sprinkle the cheese on top of the chilli and place another wholemeal wrap on top of this.
4. Once the underside is cooked, flip the quesadilla over to cook the other side (by carefully tipping it onto a large plate, then transferring this back into the pan).
5. Cut into four segments using a pizza cutter.
6. Serve with a dollop of guacamole.

Nutrition Information:

Kcal	Pro.	Fat	Sat. fat	Carb	Fibre	Added Sugar	Salt
650	29g	23g	9g	100g	18g	4g	2.5g

48. Bean burrito

Serves 1

Ingredients:
- 1 wholemeal wrap
- 3-4 tablespoons of bean chilli (see recipe for option 46. Bean chilli)
- ½ an avocado
- 1 tablespoon of natural yogurt
- 1 small handful of grated cheese (20g)
- 1 handful of spinach

Method:
1. Heat a wholemeal wrap in the microwave for a few seconds.
2. Add three to four tablespoons of bean chilli (see recipe for option 46. Bean chilli), half an avocado (sliced), one tablespoon of natural yogurt, a small handful of grated cheese, and a handful of spinach to the wrap.
3. Fold into a burrito and enjoy!

Nutrition Information:

Kcal	Pro.	Fat	Sat. fat	Carb	Fibre	Added Sugar	Salt
550	21g	33g	12g	48g	6g	5g	1.5g

49. Lentil bake

Serves 4

Ingredients:
- 2 medium onions
- 2-3 garlic cloves
- 1 tablespoon of rapeseed or olive oil
- 3 medium carrots
- 1 courgette
- 2 celery sticks
- 1 red pepper
- 1 low-salt vegetable stock cube
- 1 tin of chopped tomatoes
- 300g of split lentils
- 90g of cheese
- 200g breadcrumbs (about 6 slices of wholegrain bread crumbled up)

Method:
1. Preheat the oven to 180°C.
2. Dice the onion and garlic (or use a garlic press if you prefer) then fry these in one tablespoon of oil until the onion starts to become translucent.
3. Chop the rest of the vegetables, then add to the pan and sauté until they begin to soften.
4. Add the lentils and cover with 450ml of vegetable stock.
5. Stir in the tin of tomatoes.

6. Simmer until the lentils are cooked (you may need to add some extra boiling water to make it the consistency that you like. You can also add your favourite herbs and spices).

7. Pour the cooked lentil and vegetable mixture to an oven-proof dish, then top with breadcrumbs and grated cheese.

8. Bake for about around 20 minutes (until the cheese is golden on top).

Nutrition Information (per serving):

Kcal	Pro.	Fat	Sat. fat	Carb	Fibre	Added Sugar	Salt
580	32g	11g	5g	96g	8g	0g	1g

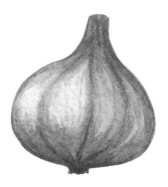

50. Tofu and sweet potato satay

Serves 4

Ingredients:
- 1 large onion
- 2-3 garlic cloves (or 1-2 teaspoons of garlic puree)
- 1 tablespoon of rapeseed oil
- 2 medium sweet potatoes
- 1 block of pressed tofu (280g)
- 3 handfuls of spinach
- 4 handfuls of frozen peas
- 4 tablespoons of peanut butter
- 1 tin of light coconut milk
- 2 tablespoons of curry powder
- 2 tablespoons of soy sauce
- 1 tablespoon of honey
- The juice of 1 lemon

Method:
1. Chop the onion and garlic and sauté with the rapeseed oil over a medium heat for two minutes.
2. While the onions are cooking, peel and chop the sweet potato into bite-sized chunks.
3. Then add the sweet potato to the pan and fry for a further five minutes until the sweet potato has started to soften.
4. Chop the tofu and add it to the pan, followed by the peas, peanut butter, soy sauce, coconut milk, honey, lemon juice and curry powder.

5. Bring this to the boil, then simmer on a low heat for ten minutes (until everything is fully cooked).
6. Then add the spinach and cook for a further minute.

Nutrition Information (per serving):

Kcal	Pro.	Fat	Sat. fat	Carb	Fibre	Added Sugar	Salt
510	20g	31g	16g	48g	10g	4g	1.4g

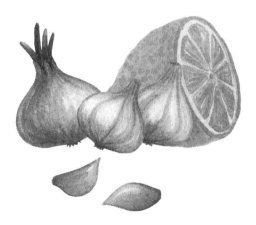

References

1. MacDonald D et al. (2018) "American Gut: an open platform for citizen-science microbe research". mSystems. [Accessed March 2020 via: https://www.ncbi.nlm.nih.gov/pubmed/29795809]

2. Scientific Advisory Committee on Nutrition (2015) "Carbohydrates and Health Report" [Accessed March 2020 via: https://www.gov.uk/government/publications/sacn-carbohydrates-and-health-report]

3. FSAI (2011) "Scientific Recommendations for Healthy Eating Guidelines in Ireland" [Accessed March 2020 via: www.fsai.ie]

4. Wu G (2016) "Dietary protein intake and human health". Food Funct. [Accessed March 2020 via: https://www.ncbi.nlm.nih.gov/pubmed/26797090]

5. Hooper L, Martin N, Abdelhamid A and Davey Smith G. (2015) "Reduction in Saturated Fat Intake For Cardiovascular Disease". Cochrane Database Syst Rev. [Accessed March 2020 via: https://www.ncbi.nlm.nih.gov/pubmed/26068959]

6. National Institute of Health (2020) "Calcium — Fact Sheet for Health Professionals". [Accessed March 2020 via: https://ods.od.nih.gov/factsheets/Calcium-HealthProfessional/]

7. National Institute of Health (2020) "Iron — Fact Sheet for Health Professionals". [Accessed March 2020 via: https://ods.od.nih.gov/factsheets/Iron-HealthProfessional/]

8. European Food Safety Authority (2011) 'Scientific

Opinion on the substantiation of health claims related to docosahexaenoic acid (DHA), eicosapentaenoic acid (EPA) and brain, eye and nerve development (ID 501, 513, 540), maintenance of normal brain function (ID 497, 501, 510, 513, 519, 521, 534, 540, 688, 1323, 1360, 4294), maintenance of normal vision (ID 508, 510, 513, 519, 529, 540, 688, 2905, 4294), maintenance of normal cardiac function (ID 510, 688, 1360)" [Accessed March 2020 via: https://efsa.onlinelibrary.wiley.com/doi/epdf/10.2903/j.efsa.2011.2078]

9. Alhassana A, Young J, Lean MEJ and Lara J (2017) "Consumption of fish and vascular risk factors: A systematic review and meta-analysis of intervention studies". Atherosclerosis. [Accessed March 2020 via: https://www.sciencedirect.com/science/article/abs/pii/S002191501731314X]

10. Roncaglioni MC, Tombesi M, Avanzini F, Barlera S, Caimi V, Longoni P, Marzona I, Milani V, Silletta MG, Tognoni G and Marchioli R (2013) "n-3 fatty acids in patients with multiple cardiovascular risk factors". N Engl J Med. [Accessed March 2020 via: https://www.ncbi.nlm.nih.gov/pubmed/23656645?dopt=Abstract]

11. Lane K, Derbyshire E, Li W andBrennan C (2014) "Bioavailability and potential uses of vegetarian sources of omega-3 fatty acids: a review of the literature". Crit Rev Food Sci Nutr. [Accessed April 2020 via: https://www.ncbi.nlm.nih.gov/pubmed/24261532]

12. Leary PF, Zamfirova I, Au J and McCracken WH (2017) "Effect of Latitude on Vitamin D Levels". J Am Osteopath Assoc. [Accessed March 2020 via: https://www.ncbi.nlm.nih.gov/pubmed/28662556]

13. Scientific Advisory Committee on Nutrition (2016) "Vitamin D and Health Report" [Accessed March 2020 via: https://assets.publishing.service.gov.uk/government/uploads/system/uploads/attachment_data/file/537616/SACN_Vitamin_D_and_Health_report.pdf]

14. National Institute of Health (2020) "Vitamin D — Fact Sheet for Health Professionals". [Accessed March 2020 via: https://ods.od.nih.gov/factsheets/VitaminD-HealthProfessional/]

15. European Food Safety Authority (2015) "Panel on Dietetic Products, Nutrition and Allergies (NDA). Safety of caffeine". EFSA Journal. [Accessed March 2020 via: https://www.efsa.europa.eu/sites/default/files/consultation/150115.pdf]

16. Drinkaware Website "UK alcohol unit guidance: CMOs' Low RiskDrinking Guidelines" [Accessed March 2020 via: https://www.drinkaware.co.uk/alcohol-facts/alcoholic-drinks-units/latest-uk-alcohol-unit-guidance/]

17. Brinkman JE & Sharma S "Physiology, Body Fluids" [Accessed April 2020 via: https://www.ncbi.nlm.nih.gov/books/NBK482447/]

18. British Dietetic Association "Fluid (water and drinks): Food Fact Sheet" [Accessed March 2020 via: https://www.bda.uk.com/resource/fluid-water-drinks.html]

19. Harandi TF, Taghinasab MM, and Nayeri TD (2017) "The correlation of social support with mental health: A meta-analysis". Electron Physician. [Accessed March 2020 via: https://www.ncbi.nlm.nih.gov/pmc/articles/PMC56332

15/]

20. Hsiao YH, Chang CH and Gean PW (2018) "Impact of social relationships on Alzheimer's memory impairment: mechanistic studies". J Biomed Sci. [Accessed March 2020 via: https://www.ncbi.nlm.nih.gov/pmc/articles/PMC5764000/]

21. Umberson D and Montez JK (2010) "Social Relationships and Health: A Flashpoint for Health Policy". J Health Soc Behav. [Accessed March 2020 via: https://www.ncbi.nlm.nih.gov/pmc/articles/PMC3150158/]

22. Regulation (EU) No 1169/2011 on the provision of food information to consumers, amending Regulations (EC) No 1924/2006 and (EC) No 1925/2006 of the European Parliament and of the Council, and repealing Commission Directive 87/250/EEC, Council Directive 90/496/EEC, Commission Directive 1999/10/EC, Directive 2000/13/EC of the European Parliament and of the Council, Commission Directives 2002/67/EC and 2008/5/EC and Commission Regulation (EC) No 608/2004 [Accessed March 2020 via: https://eur-lex.europa.eu/legal-content/EN/TXT/?uri=CELEX:02011R1169-20180101]

23. Jiménez-Monreal AM, García-Diz L, Martínez-Tomé M, Mariscal M and Murcia MA (2009) "Influence of cooking methods on antioxidant activity of vegetables". J Food Sci. [Accessed March 2020 via: https://www.ncbi.nlm.nih.gov/pubmed/19397724]

24. FSA "Cooking and Reheating Safely" [Accessed March 2020 via: https://www.food.gov.uk/sites/default/files/media/document/sfbb-childminders-cooking-reheating.pdf]

25. NHS Website "Reference intakes explained" (2017) [Accessed March 2020 via: https://www.nhs.uk/live-well/eat-well/what-are-reference-intakes-on-food-labels/]

26. IntuitiveEating.org "10 Principles of Intuitive Eating" [Accessed May 2020 via: https://www.intuitiveeating.org/10-principles-of-intuitive-eating/]

27. HPRA (2018) "Medical Devices Information Notice: Food Intolerance Testing" [Accessed April 2020 via: https://www.indi.ie/images/HPRA_Medical-devices-information-note_on_food_intolerance_testing.pdf]

28. NHS Website (2019) "Exercise" [Accessed March 2020 via: https://www.nhs.uk/live-well/exercise/]

29. NHS Website (2018) "Why lack of sleep is bad for your health" [Accessed March 2020 via: https://www.nhs.uk/live-well/sleep-and-tiredness/why-lack-of-sleep-is-bad-for-your-health/]

30. Drinkaware Website "Health Effects of Alcohol" [Accessed March 2020 via: https://www.drinkaware.co.uk/alcohol-facts/health-effects-of-alcohol/]

31. NHS Website "How smoking affects your body" [Accessed March 2020 via: https://www.nhs.uk/smokefree/why-quit/smoking-health-problems

Printed in Great Britain
by Amazon